To my husband Gordon,
thanks for being so supportive

Acknowledgements

I'd like to thank Jennifer Barclay for commissioning this book and for helping me to organise the information. I'd also like to thank Alice Theadom for taking time out of her busy schedule to write the foreword. Thanks also to Emily Kearns and Chris Turton for their useful editorial input.

Other titles in the Personal Health Guides series include:

50 Things You Can Do Today to Increase Your Fertility
50 Things You Can Do Today to Manage Anxiety
50 Things You Can Do Today to Manage Arthritis
50 Things You Can Do Today to Manage Back Pain
50 Things You Can Do Today to Manage Eczema
50 Things You Can Do Today to Manage Hay Fever
50 Things You Can Do Today to Manage IBS
50 Things You Can Do Today to Manage Insomnia
50 Things You Can Do Today to Manage Migraines
50 Things You Can Do Today to Manage Menopause
50 Things You Can Do Today to Manage Stress

50 things you can do today to manage
today to manage
fibromyalgia

Foreword by Alice Theadom,
Senior Research Fellow at the National Institute for
Stroke and Applied Neuroscience, AUT University

Wendy Green

PERSONAL HEALTH GUIDES

50 THINGS YOU CAN DO TODAY TO MANAGE FIBROMYALGIA

Summersdale Publishers Ltd
46 West Street
Chichester
West Sussex
PO19 1RP
UK

www.summersdale.com

Printed and bound in the UK by CPI Group (UK) Ltd, Croydon, CR0 4YY

ISBN: 978-1-84953-203-7

Substantial discounts on bulk quantities of Summersdale books are available to corporations, professional associations and other organisations. For details contact Summersdale Publishers by telephone: +44 (0) 1243 771107, fax: +44 (0) 1243 786300 or email: nicky@summersdale.com.

Disclaimer
Every effort has been made to ensure that the information in this book is accurate and current at the time of publication. The author and the publisher cannot accept responsibility for any misuse or misunderstanding of any information contained herein, or any loss, damage or injury, be it health, financial or otherwise, suffered by any individual or group acting upon or relying on information contained herein. None of the opinions or suggestions in this book is intended to replace medical opinion. If you have concerns about your health, please seek professional advice.

Contents

1. Learn about fibromyalgia
2. Identify your triggers

3. Keep a stress diary
4. Try the ABC of CBT
5. Pace yourself
6. Clear away clutter
7. Try not to worry
8. Live in the moment
9. Assert yourself
10. Find support
11. Laugh more
12. Get closer to nature
13. Practise relaxation techniques

Author's Note

While I don't have fibromyalgia, I do suffer from chronic pain in my neck and shoulders, so I know only too well how difficult it is to live with constant pain. I also suffer from IBS and migraines from time to time, so again, this gives me some insight into how it feels to have fibromyalgia. However, I can't begin to imagine what it must be like to suffer from a myriad of other symptoms as well – especially the constant fatigue and exhaustion that is part and parcel of fibromyalgia syndrome.

While the condition is not life-threatening, it can be so debilitating that taking part in normal, everyday activities is virtually impossible. As is the case for most health conditions, there is no magical formula that will work for everyone, so I have included in these 50 things a variety of alternative and conventional approaches, in the sincere hope that every reader will find effective ways to help them manage their individual symptoms.

Wendy Green

Foreword

by Alice Theadom,
Senior Research Fellow at the National Institute for
Stroke and Applied Neuroscience, AUT University

Over the ten years that I have been working with people with fibromyalgia, knowledge of the condition has grown immensely. In many of my first discussions with clinicians, few recognised fibromyalgia as a legitimate condition, let alone knew how to treat it. Now, although there may remain debate about the most accurate method of diagnosis, the triggers and the best treatment approach, fibromyalgia is a recognised condition and research evidence is rapidly growing.

The onset of fibromyalgia can change the lives of those affected and the people around them in so many ways. As this book eloquently describes, people's experiences of fibromyalgia can be very different. For example, for some people symptoms appear gradually, whereas for others, symptoms can occur suddenly following a 'life event', such as childbirth or an accident/illness. The range of symptoms as a result of the condition can also vary considerably. It has therefore been encouraging to see the recent emergence of treatment guidelines that emphasise the need for an individual approach to treatment, rather than the previous one-size-fits-all approach that focused only on the treatment of pain.

It is based on this holistic view of fibromyalgia, that this book offers strategies that may help people to identify their own personal triggers, in addition to ideas to help manage the condition. The author's easy-to-read style and possible explanations of how the strategies might work, encourage the reader to identify those that may be most suitable for them. Research evidence is presented where available, although it is clear that much more research is needed to answer many of the remaining questions about fibromyalgia. With the wide range of strategies presented and an overview of information on fibromyalgia, it is hoped there is something in this book for everyone.

Introduction

Up until the last decade or so, fibromyalgia was not widely recognised by the medical profession. Many people who suffered from persistent widespread pain, and other physical and psychological symptoms, were told they had arthritis or rheumatism and were perhaps prescribed painkillers. However, in recent years research has shed light on the condition and many more GPs now recognise the symptoms. Even so, the condition is not included in the National Institute for Health and Clinical Excellence (NICE) guidelines, which means some GPs still do not have a clear understanding of the symptoms and how best to treat them. This means it is often difficult for a person suffering from fibromyalgia to get a firm diagnosis and appropriate treatment.

This book will help you to understand the condition and enable you to work with your GP to find the best ways to manage it. While there is no outright cure for fibromyalgia, dramatic improvements can be achieved through self-help measures – such as those outlined in this book; organisations that provide information and support to fibromyalgia sufferers in the UK, such as FibroAction, the Fibromyalgia Association UK and UK Fibromyalgia all recommend sufferers take an active role in their treatment by adopting self-management techniques.

This book explains what fibromyalgia is and outlines the wide range of symptoms sufferers may experience. It looks at the psychological, physical, nutritional, biological and environmental factors that may be involved in the development of this complex condition, and offers a holistic approach and practical advice to help you manage your symptoms.

There is a section covering cognitive behavioural therapy (CBT) techniques, which involve adopting a more positive attitude, and other behaviours that have been shown to help sufferers to cope. You will discover how to listen to your body, so you pace yourself and know when to rest to avoid flare-ups. Relaxation and stress-management techniques, such as meditation, deep breathing, creative visualisation and muscle relaxation, are included. You will learn how gentle exercise can help to ease pain, and discover the benefits of activities such as walking and yoga.

You will also find out which foods provide the nutrients that may help to prevent or relieve your symptoms. There is an overview of the dietary supplements that may assist in the easing of symptoms such as pain, fatigue, depression and poor sleep. Everyday life can be difficult when you have fibromyalgia, so there are practical tips to help you cope with flare-ups and activities like household chores, driving, working and travelling. There is also advice on how to deal with insomnia, migraines, irritable bowel syndrome (IBS), restless legs syndrome (RLS) and Raynaud's, which are frequently part of the fibromyalgia syndrome.

It is likely that at some point you will need to consider taking one or more of the medications currently used for the treatment of fibromyalgia, so there is an overview of those most commonly used. There's also a selection of relaxing and pain-relieving techniques and treatments from complementary therapies you can try for yourself. At the end of the book you'll find recipes based on the dietary guidelines, as well as details of helpful products, books and organisations.

Chapter 1

About Fibromyalgia

This chapter explains what fibromyalgia is and gives an overview of the symptoms. It also considers the psychological, physical, nutritional, biological and environmental factors that may contribute to the development of fibromyalgia. The chapter ends with two fibromyalgia sufferer's stories and advice on identifying your triggers.

1. Learn about fibromyalgia

What is fibromyalgia?

Fibromyalgia, formerly known as fibrositis or rheumatism, is a debilitating, chronic (long-term) condition that is thought to affect up to 1.8 million people in the UK. The word 'fibromyalgia' means 'tendon, ligament and muscle pain' but sufferers usually experience a variety of additional symptoms.

Flare-ups of the condition can last for several days, weeks or months. Although fibromyalgia is not a type of arthritis, as it doesn't affect the joints, some arthritis sufferers do go on to develop it. Women are more likely to suffer from fibromyalgia than men, as are those aged 50 to 70 – although it can sometimes affect children and young people as well. With appropriate management and treatment, people with mild to moderate fibromyalgia can usually lead a normal life; however, if symptoms are severe, the sufferer may be unable to work or have an active social life. Another problem is that because sufferers often look well, other people may find it hard to appreciate the pain and debilitation fibromyalgia causes.

What are the symptoms of fibromyalgia?

Fibromyalgia is a syndrome that consists of a collection of symptoms mainly involving widespread pain and tenderness in the muscles, ligaments and tendons in various parts of the body, such as the arms, legs, neck and back. The pain may vary in intensity and can be worse in certain areas of the body, e.g. your back or neck. It is usually continuous and can be anything from an ache or a burning sensation – some describe it as feeling like 'burning acid' – to a sharp, stabbing pain, while some experts have recently suggested it feels like 'a thousand needles'. The pain can stem from a variety of sources including muscular tension, poor muscular strength, muscular stiffness and 'trigger points'. Trigger points (not tender points) are areas where the muscles are taut, knotted and painful. When a trigger point is activated in some way, perhaps through stress, exertion or the cold, it transmits pain or numbness to other areas of the body. For example, if you press on a trigger point at the base of your neck, you might feel pain or numbness down one arm. Trigger point massage can help to relax the muscle and relieve the pain (see Action 49 – Massage away pain).

The condition can make you so sensitive to pain (hyperalgesia) that you find even the lightest touch painful (allodynia), or if you hurt yourself you might find that the pain continues for longer than normal. Despite causing a lot of pain, however, fibromyalgia doesn't cause permanent damage to the muscles, bones or joints.

What is pain?

Put simply, pain is a warning message to the brain that there is something wrong with the body. Nerve cells in the skin and tissues detect when you suffer an injury, and chemicals called neurotransmitters communicate this information via nerve pathways to the spinal cord, which transmits the message on to the brain. Your perception of pain can be affected by your mood at the time and even your beliefs about pain, as well as past experiences of it. So pain is not a straightforward response to injury or damage, it is also an emotional one; if you are tense, unhappy or frightened you may interpret pain as more severe than if you are feeling relaxed and happy.

In acute pain, once the injury has healed, the pain receptors no longer detect any damage and the pain stops. However, when there is long-term damage – such as that caused by arthritis – the nerve cells will continue to transmit pain messages to the brain; this is known as chronic pain. The pain of fibromyalgia is not thought to be due to long-term tissue damage, although it can sometimes be triggered by an injury, as the pain continues long after the injury has healed. Therefore experts believe that fibromyalgia pain is due to an oversensitive nervous system, perhaps caused by imbalances in chemicals involved in pain transmission.

Other symptoms include:

Stiffness – this can be more severe when you have been in the same position for a long time, e.g. when you wake up in the morning.

Muscular spasm – this is where the muscles contract tightly, causing pain, which can cause problems with sleeping.

Sleep disturbances – it is thought that the pain of fibromyalgia makes sleeping difficult. You may not get enough deep sleep, so you wake up feeling tired even when you think you have had plenty of sleep.

Extreme fatigue – this can range from feeling tired to experiencing flu-like exhaustion. It can come on quickly, leaving sufferers drained of energy. Some sufferers report feeling as though their arms and legs are weighed down by concrete blocks. Sleep disturbances can contribute to the fatigue.

Irritability, anxiety and depression – it is not clear whether these symptoms are part of the syndrome, or if they are due to the pain, lack of sleep and fatigue.

Cognitive problems ('fibro-fog') – these are difficulties with thinking and learning, such as poor concentration and memory, and mixing up words.

Headaches – suffering from pain and stiffness in your neck and shoulders from fibromyalgia can trigger mild headaches to more severe migraines.

Tinnitus – a ringing or other sound in your ears or head that is not due to external noise.

Irritable bowel syndrome (IBS) – some fibromyalgia sufferers also develop IBS, a common digestive condition that causes tummy pain, bloating, constipation and diarrhoea.

Irritable bladder – you may need to go to the toilet to pass urine more often.

Sensitivity to certain foods, bright lights, noise, temperature (Raynaud's phenomenon), smoke, chemicals – exposure to something you are sensitive to can trigger a flare-up.

Restless legs syndrome (RLS) – the symptoms of RLS are 'creeping or crawling' sensations in your legs that cause you to move them around to find relief.

How is fibromyalgia diagnosed?

A recent European survey found that it takes around 18 months to two years to be diagnosed with fibromyalgia. The condition is often difficult to detect because there is no specific test and the symptoms can resemble those of other illnesses, such as chronic fatigue syndrome, multiple sclerosis, lupus, Lyme disease and rheumatoid arthritis; your GP may carry out tests to rule these conditions out. Another problem is that many GPs treat each symptom individually, because they fail to recognise they are all part of one condition.

For your GP to be able to make a firm diagnosis you should have experienced the pain continuously for at least three months. The pain and tenderness should be widespread, affecting both sides of the body above and below the waist; your GP may carry out the 'tender point test' – which involves applying light pressure to 18 specific sites on the neck, shoulders, elbows, chest, lower back and knees. Pain and tenderness in at least 11 of these sites is an indication that you have fibromyalgia.

Your GP may refer you to a rheumatologist (a doctor who specialises in rheumatic and arthritic conditions), who may carry out tests to check whether you have a rheumatic disease. You may also be referred to a pain clinic, where doctors specialising in pain management can diagnose the condition and offer suitable treatments.

What causes fibromyalgia?

Rather than having one specific cause, research suggests that various factors may contribute to fibromyalgia, including:

Psychological

☐ Chronic stress/tension

☐ Depression

☐ Emotional traumas, such as divorce or bereavement

☐ Repressed emotions

Physical

☐ Accidents

☐ Injuries

☐ Surgery

◯ Bad posture

◯ Over-exertion

Nutritional

◯ Nutritional deficiencies

◯ Food intolerances

◯ Caffeine

◯ Alcohol

Biological

◯ Viral or bacterial infections triggering an abnormal immune response

◯ Over-sensitive central nervous system, i.e. hypersensitivity to pain, light and noise; fibromyalgia is sometimes described as a 'central sensitisation syndrome'

◯ Low levels of neurotransmitters, such as serotonin, the 'happy hormone'

◯ Higher-than-normal levels of substance P, a chemical involved in the transmission of pain in the body

◯ Low levels of cortisol, a hormone released by the adrenal glands in response to stress

- Low levels of growth hormone, which is released by the pituitary gland

- Rheumatoid arthritis, osteoarthritis and lupus – you may be more likely to develop fibromyalgia if you suffer from one of these conditions

- Hypothyroidism (underactive thyroid)

- Gender – fibromyalgia affects ten times as many women as men, possibly because of hormonal fluctuations, e.g. before a menstrual period and during the menopause

- Age – the condition mainly affects older people

- Genetics – the syndrome can run in families

- Sleep problems – may be both a cause and effect of fibromyalgia, and can have both physical and psychological causes

Environmental

- Toxin overload from car fumes, food additives, chemicals found in toiletries and cleaning products etc

- Changes in the weather

- Exposure to cold or draughts

Two fibromyalgia sufferers' stories

Every fibromyalgia sufferer will have their own individual triggers and symptoms, and can discover what lifestyle changes and treatments work best for them. Below are two fibromyalgia sufferers' stories.

Eileen, 59

Eileen, a nurse, has suffered from fibromyalgia for 13 years. She describes her main symptoms as pain and discomfort in her upper arms and legs, which causes weakness, stiffness upon waking and general fatigue. Eileen was already seeing her GP about chronic fatigue when her fibromyalgia symptoms developed. Her GP diagnosed fibromyalgia within about six to nine months and prescribed the painkillers Voltarol and Tramadol to control the pain. Eileen says: 'My GP didn't offer me any advice, but I think he was aware I had done my own research into how to manage the condition.'

She has found over the years that stressful situations such as family illness or bereavement can trigger a flare-up. She says: 'I've noticed that eating acidic foods, and drinking coffee and alcohol, can make my symptoms worse.'

Suffering from fibromyalgia has changed her lifestyle quite dramatically. She comments: 'Prior to suffering from fibromyalgia I was very active. I had a physical job as a staff nurse in palliative cancer day care at a local hospice and I loved to keep fit, dancing, gardening and decorating. Now I am severely restricted in what I can do.'

However, Eileen has found that changing her job and working fewer hours, combined with pacing herself, has helped her to live with the condition. She explains: 'I have changed jobs and now work part-time in health promotion, carrying out health screening and giving general health advice. I also alternate between doing physical and mental activities. I only do anything physical, such as housework, for ten to 15 minutes. After that I rest or do paperwork, or some other mental activity.'

Eileen has found that the prescribed painkillers, combined with paracetamol, help to ease the pain. She adds: 'I've found vitamin B complex helps to ease my symptoms. I also used to find capsaicin gel helped a lot with the pain, but it was difficult to manage regular applications, so I stopped using it.' She finds relaxation helps, too – especially meditation.

Maria, 34

Maria, a writer, was just 28 years old when she began experiencing sharp, shooting pains in her hands. At first she thought she was suffering from repetitive strain injury (RSI), due to the long hours she was spending using a computer keyboard, both in her day job with a publisher and in the course of forging a career as a writer. She thought she would be fine if she rested her hands, but her condition rapidly worsened. She says the pain she felt was 'as if the blood in my hands was poisoned with burning acid'. Within a week, the pain spread to her arms and legs. 'It was like a nightmare,' she recalls. 'I couldn't sleep because of the pain and even a short walk was agony. I was only 28, but I felt like an old woman.'

She went to see her GP, who applied pressure to various areas on her body. Maria says: 'When he pressed the base of my neck, I nearly jumped out of my seat with the pain.' Her GP also carried out blood tests to check for conditions such as rheumatoid arthritis. He eventually diagnosed fibromyalgia and told her it was a chronic pain condition that would never go away, but she could learn to manage it.

Maria was prescribed strong painkillers and amitriptyline, an anti-depressant sometimes used for sleeping problems. She remembers feeling distraught: 'I didn't want to be ill for the rest of my life. And what would happen to my dream of becoming an author if I couldn't use a computer keyboard?'

After reading on a fibromyalgia forum that you need to attack the condition head-on, she decided to do all she could to tackle her symptoms. She began noticing that certain foods, including wheat and refined sugars, and alcohol, seemed to make the pain worse; so, under her GP's supervision, she cut these out of her diet. After a few weeks the pain began to lessen. She also had acupuncture treatments, and took multivitamins, magnesium and ginseng to help beat fatigue, and melatonin to help regulate her sleep. She also began walking, gradually building up to 40 minutes a day. The pain started to ease 'from red-hot to a severe ache'.

She eventually built up enough energy to return to work, but there were times when she was so tired she couldn't even get out of bed. It was three years before she felt well enough to stop taking the amitriptyline. She is now more or less pain-free, but realises if she overdoes things, or doesn't get enough sleep, the nasty tingling in her arms and legs will return.

What can you do to manage fibromyalgia?

These two case studies demonstrate that the symptoms of fibromyalgia can be devastating, but that with careful management, including making sure you pace yourself, it is still possible to lead a fulfilling life.

The first and most obvious place to start when aiming to manage your condition is to identify what triggers a flare-up.

2. Identify your triggers

The best way to identify what triggers your fibromyalgia flare-ups is to keep a diary in which you record details of your symptoms and everyday life, including your diet, sleep and physical activity patterns, as well as any situations you are finding stressful. Over a period of time you should start noticing a pattern emerging.

Once you have pinpointed your triggers, you can start adapting your lifestyle to take control of your symptoms. For example, if you find that your symptoms reappear, or get worse, if you don't eat well, or if you overdo things or don't get enough sleep, this might involve improving your diet, pacing yourself and practising good sleep hygiene. Other strategies that may help you deal with fibromyalgia include taking gentle exercise, following relaxation techniques, trying complementary therapies, managing stress and adopting a positive attitude.

This book aims to offer you practical advice in all of these areas to help you both prevent and relieve your fibromyalgia symptoms.

Chapter 2

Pace Yourself, Rest and Relax

Pacing, resting and relaxing are ways of planning your life to help you to avoid overdoing things, reduce stress and replenish energy levels, thereby preventing painful flare-ups and relieving fatigue.

Many fibromyalgia sufferers report that their symptoms start, or are made worse, after a period of stress. In this chapter we initially look at what stress is, the effects it has on the body and how it might be both a cause and effect of fibromyalgia flare-ups.

We then look at ways of managing stress, such as avoiding your stressors, thinking positively and simplifying your life by pacing yourself and listening to your body, to avoid overdoing things. We also consider other proven stress-management strategies, such as living in the present, being assertive and engaging with nature.

Rest and relaxation can help fibromyalgia, not only by reducing stress but also by relieving fatigue and loosening the muscles, thereby reducing pain; at the end of the chapter you will find some relaxation techniques including meditation, deep breathing, creative visualisation and muscle relaxation.

Techniques like these are collectively known as cognitive behavioural therapy (CBT). CBT is a type of psychotherapy that targets thinking and behaviour patterns to relieve health issues, such as stress and chronic pain. A study funded by Arthritis Research UK in 2011 involving 442 fibromyalgia sufferers found that 30 per cent of those who received TCBT (CBT over the telephone) reported an improvement in their symptoms, including fatigue, sleep problems and overall well-being, after six months, with 33 per cent still noticing improvements after nine months; this study illustrates that taking control of your thoughts and behaviour can play a huge part in managing your symptoms.

What is stress?

In a nutshell, stress is the way the mind and body respond to situations and pressures that leave us feeling inadequate, or unable to cope. One person may cope well in a situation that another might find stressful; it's all down to the individual's perception of it and their ability to deal with it. If you have to cope with debilitating fibromyalgia symptoms, it is likely that you will find dealing with many other aspects of everyday life that healthy individuals take in their stride – such as holding down a job, doing domestic chores and enjoying a social life – very stressful.

How does stress affect the body?

The brain responds to stress by preparing the body to either face the perceived threat, or to escape from it. It does this by releasing hormones – chemical messengers – such as adrenaline, noradrenaline and cortisol, into the bloodstream. These speed up the heart rate and breathing patterns, and can induce sweating. Glucose and fatty acid levels in the blood rise to provide a burst of energy to deal with the threat. This is called the 'fight or flight' response.

Today the events that trigger the stress response are unlikely to necessitate either of these reactions. Those that go on for a long period of time with no end in sight, for example, chronic illness, long-term unemployment or an unhappy relationship, cause stress hormone levels to remain high, thereby increasing the risk of major health conditions, such as coronary heart disease and stroke, as well as autoimmune disorders, such as rheumatoid arthritis. Other psychological and physical symptoms include irritability, poor concentration, anxiety, depression, headaches, skin problems, allergies, poor appetite or overeating, indigestion, IBS and heart palpitations.

How is stress involved in fibromyalgia symptoms?

Many people develop fibromyalgia after a stressful period in their lives, but how can stress be involved in fibromyalgia symptoms? It seems that the answer lies in the chemical processes that take place in the body during the stress response.

Researchers believe that stress hormones such as cortisol affect the balance of cytokines, a type of white blood cell produced within the central nervous system that is involved in the immune response. After a while, levels of Th1 cytokines are lowered, which leaves the body more prone to infections, while Th2 cytokine levels are raised; higher levels of Th2 cytokines are linked to inflammation and increased allergic and autoimmune responses. Several studies have found that fibromyalgia sufferers often have above-average levels of these inflammatory cytokines and that the higher the levels are, the greater the intensity of pain experienced.

Stressed people often suffer from sleep problems – which are also thought to be involved in the development of fibromyalgia. Also, when people are stressed they often turn to junk food, caffeine, alcohol and nicotine to help them cope – all of which can lead to the nutritional deficiencies that may be linked to fibromyalgia. Clearly, managing stress is an important part of taking control of your fibromyalgia symptoms.

What can I do about stress?

There are basically three things you can do to manage stress: avoid it, reduce it and relieve it.

3. Keep a stress diary

For a couple of weeks note down the details of situations, times, places and people that make you feel stressed. Once you've identified these, think about each one and ask yourself: 'Can I avoid this?' For example, if you find going shopping at the supermarket stressful, perhaps you could shop online instead.

If you cannot avoid a particular stressor, you can usually reduce the level of stress you experience by taking practical steps to help you cope better, such as eating well (see Chapter 4 – Eat Foods That Fight Fibromyalgia), taking exercise (see Chapter 3 – Exercise to Ease Pain) and getting plenty of sleep (see Chapter 6 – Live Better With Fibromyalgia), or by changing your attitude towards the situation. You can reduce your overall stress levels by simplifying your life, in particular by pacing yourself, prioritising and learning to focus more on the present.

You can also relieve the effects of stress by taking time out for yourself, practising relaxation techniques and doing things that help you unwind.

4. Try the ABC of CBT

Often it is not a situation itself that is stressful but how we perceive it. Changing a negative mindset to a positive one can totally change the way we view events.

For example, you don't hear from a friend for several weeks and automatically assume they want to end your friendship, so you don't contact them. If you viewed this from a more positive angle you might think of other reasons why your friend didn't contact you, for example, they were too busy, or they were ill, and decide to give them a call.

Cognitive behavioural therapy (CBT) is a type of psychotherapy that focuses on replacing negative thoughts and unhelpful behaviours, which can lead to emotional issues – including stress – with more positive ones. It works on the underlying principle that your thoughts affect your feelings, your feelings affect your actions and your actions come full circle to affect your thoughts again. According to cognitive theory, many of us develop negative beliefs about ourselves as a result of our experiences during childhood and early adulthood, e.g. being bullied at school, parents divorcing, failing an exam, etc., and these take root in our minds until they become automatic. Behavioural theory is based on the belief that behaviour is a learned response that is also a reaction to past experiences. CBT is based on both principles.

According to CBT your feelings aren't facts – they are just your perception of an event or situation. In other words, an event or situation is only as stressful as you think it is. Your perception of events in your life and how you respond to them is down to the filters through which you look at them. These filters include your personality, values, beliefs and attitudes, which have been shaped by your genetics, upbringing, past experiences, lifestyle and culture. It is possible to change your perception of an event, and your subsequent behaviour, simply by changing your beliefs about yourself and situations.

Try the ABC approach next time you're feeling stressed:

Activator – note down the situation that triggered your stress, e.g. being diagnosed with fibromyalgia.

Beliefs – list your thoughts about the situation, e.g. 'I won't be able to cope with the pain', 'I won't be able to manage everyday tasks.'

Consequences of A plus B – record your feelings and actions, e.g. worried, apprehensive, frightened, tense muscles.

Dispute your negative thoughts – that is, identify alternative, positive ways of viewing the situation, e.g. 'I've been dealing with the pain for a while, so I know I can cope', 'Now that I know what I am suffering from I can take positive steps to take control of my symptoms.'

Effective new approaches – choose new, helpful behaviours, e.g. 'I'll make a list of realistic changes I can make to my lifestyle to help manage my symptoms', 'I'll ask my family and friends to help me with tasks I can't manage on my own'.

If you follow this formula each time you face difficulties, you will gradually build a more positive image of yourself and your ability to cope with whatever life throws at you. This will give you the confidence to find effective solutions and reduce the amount of stress you experience.

Abandon perfectionism

As well as recognising the external factors that make you feel stressed, consider whether some aspects of your personality are also to blame. Are you a perfectionist with high expectations of yourself, perhaps based on what you could do when you were well, which you can no longer achieve? Constantly feeling that who you are and what you have aren't good enough can lead to discontent and worry – unnecessary pressure that can lead to tension and increased pain.

To make life easier for yourself, stop thinking about what you could do in the past and focus on what you can realistically hope to achieve now. This will necessitate pacing yourself, which involves listening to your body to find out what you can do each day, alternating periods of work with rest, following a routine, and prioritising tasks.

5. Pace yourself

Pacing yourself means alternating periods of activity with periods of rest. It requires you to listen to your body so that you don't do too much or push yourself beyond your limits.

Listen to your body

Remember how Action 2 – Identify your triggers suggested that you should record details of your symptoms and everyday life, including your physical activity patterns? This information can also help you to pace yourself. Read through your diary and see if you can identify:

1. How much physical and mental activity you can handle each day.

2. Which activities you find the most taxing.

3. The times of day you have the most energy.

4. Your 'early warning signs' that indicate you are reaching your limit – e.g. pain or tingling in your hands, or extreme fatigue.

Once you know the answers to these questions you are ready to start pacing yourself.

Work in short bursts

If you have a big task to do, don't try to complete it all in one go. Instead alternate short bursts of work with short breaks.

The length of time you spend working and resting depends on how much activity you can cope with in one go. It's usually best to err on the side of caution and start with shorter periods than you think you can handle, and rest for at least 15 minutes in between. Monitor how you feel for a couple of days, then tweak the times until you find the right balance. If you start experiencing your early warning signs always take a short break from whatever you are doing if you can.

Alternate between physical and mental tasks

Rather than doing one type of activity for a long time, try to alternate between physical and mental tasks, so that you don't overtax your muscles or drain your physical and mental energy.

For example, if you need to change the bedding, vacuum, check your bank account and respond to emails, don't do them in that order! Instead, you could perhaps change the bedding first, then check your bank account, vacuum, then answer your emails. By alternating between physical and mental activities, you avoid overworking your muscles and your brain. Don't forget that you may need to take short breaks in between each activity, too. Avoid doing any activity that pushes you too hard.

> ### Ask for help
>
> Don't assume that you should always have to do everything yourself. When you feel overloaded with tasks, ask for help. Ask your partner and children to help with household chores. Don't be too proud to accept offers of help from colleagues at work.

Take time out

As well as taking short breaks in between activities, aim to fit in one or two rest periods a day if you can, as these can really make a difference to your energy levels. Your rest periods could involve lying down and resting, taking a short nap (i.e. no more than 30 minutes in the early afternoon, to avoid disrupting sleep at night), soaking in a warm bath, or doing some deep breathing or meditating (see Action 13 – Practise relaxation techniques). The length of time you spend relaxing obviously depends on your needs and circumstances, but even 30 minutes could give you a boost. Make sure you rest both your mind and body – checking your emails, reading the newspaper, writing a shopping list or watching TV don't count as resting!

Stick to a routine

Try to stick to a steady level of activity all of the time to avoid overdoing things. Having a routine for household chores, and at work if possible, can help a lot with pacing, as it means you can slot in just one or two heavy activities each day – depending on your personal limits – rather than ending up with a lot of heavy tasks to do at once. However, bear in mind that you will still need to be flexible; on a good day you might fit in one extra task, while on a bad day you may have to just leave everything and catch up later on, when you feel better. This will involve prioritising what needs to be done first, so that you don't end up feeling overwhelmed and exhausted.

> ### Use a traffic light system
>
> Use a weekly planner to schedule in activities using a traffic light system. Mark those activities you find easy and enjoyable with a green highlighter pen, those you find a little more taxing with a yellow pen, and those you find difficult and tiring with a red pen. Avoid having too many 'red' and 'yellow' activities planned for the same day.

Prioritise

Prioritising is an important aspect of pacing. Start by having a clear sense of what you need to get done each day. Writing a 'to-do' list can help you to achieve this. When you have a long 'to-do' list, divide it into three sections:

1. **Needs** – tasks that you must do that day otherwise there will be consequences to deal with. For example, paying household bills or going food shopping. Make sure you do these first – but remember to work in short bursts, alternate tasks and take breaks.

2. **Wants** – activities you would like to do if you have the energy. For example, meeting a friend for coffee. Schedule these in

if you can, as they are usually things that contribute to your general happiness and satisfaction with life.

3. **Shoulds** – things that you do because you feel you ought to, for example, visiting an elderly relative. When you're feeling unwell you may have to say 'no' to non-essential tasks. If you feel guilty about saying 'no' it might help the other person to understand if you explain the constraints of your illness and promise to do whatever it is later, when you are feeling better. You might also consider brushing up on your assertiveness skills (see Action 9 – Assert yourself).

6. Clear away clutter

If a bulging wardrobe, heaving shelves and overflowing cupboards are getting you down, make your life simpler and less stressful by getting rid of unnecessary clutter around your home. You'll save time and energy, because your home will be easier to keep clean and tidy, and you'll find things more quickly in a clutter-free environment; your mental clarity will also improve, because ridding yourself of physical clutter clears the mind.

If you haven't worn, read or used an item for two years or more, give it to a charity shop, sell it on eBay or bin it. If you can't bear to get rid of it, store it in the loft – then make it a rule that if you haven't thought about using the item within six months, it is time to part with it. If you have a lot of possessions to sort out, ask your partner, a family member or a friend to help you. Remember to pace yourself – don't attempt to clear the whole house in one go. Break it down into areas and give yourself plenty of time to complete each one, e.g.

empty the bathroom cupboard one week, a wardrobe another week. You'll be amazed at how much happier and less stressed you will feel after a good clear out.

7. Try not to worry

Worrying about events that haven't even happened can bring on the stress response, as your body can't differentiate between what has actually happened and what you imagine might happen. For example, if you fear that your fibromyalgia might get worse, or you worry about paying your mortgage, your body will produce stress hormones, even if your condition doesn't actually deteriorate, or you don't lose your home. Although it's hard not to worry about the things that might go wrong in your life, it's better for your health if you can make a conscious decision not to worry about things that haven't happened yet. Living in the present is far less stressful.

8. Live in the moment

Living in the moment, or practising mindfulness, has been shown to reduce stress levels. It involves giving all of your attention to the here and now, rather than worrying about the past or future. It has its roots in Buddhism and is based on the philosophy that you can't alter the past, or foretell the future, but you can influence what's happening in your life right now. By living fully in the present, you can perform to the best of your ability and take pleasure from what is happening around you, whereas worrying about the past or future, or daydreaming, can hamper how you function now and increase your stress levels unnecessarily; this in turn creates tension, which can exacerbate pain.

Living in the present means making the most of every moment as it unfolds, appreciating everything around you – the colour and scent of a flower, the taste and smell of your favourite food… When you focus on the here and now, you will find yourself enjoying the simple things in your life more. Living in this way means your experience of life is richer, because instead of doing things on autopilot, all of your senses will be fully engaged in what you are doing. Think of how much you can miss when your thoughts are elsewhere instead of making the most of now.

On a more practical level, if you focus on the task in hand instead of worrying about other jobs you need to do, you are likely to complete it faster and more efficiently. If you don't have a lot of time to spend with your partner, family or friends, focusing completely on them when you are together, rather than thinking about or doing other things at the same time, will be far more rewarding for everyone.

Living in the present is a skill that can be learnt. Don't worry if you find it difficult at first – whenever you notice your mind wandering, bring it back to the here and now. Yoga involves focusing on your breathing and your body as you carry out different postures, and is a good way to practice living in the moment. The Alexander technique also encourages you to concentrate on the present by teaching you how to become more aware of your body, how you hold yourself and how you move. Doing a physical activity like swimming, or something you find absorbing like cooking a meal, painting a picture, knitting or sewing, can also bring you 'back' to the present. Keeping a daily diary can help, too, because it encourages you to think about what has happened in your life today.

Try this:

- When you're eating, focus on the sight, smell, taste and texture of your food – don't watch TV or read at the same time.

- When you're having a conversation, actively listen to what the other person is saying, instead of letting your mind wander.

- When you're doing a chore, such as washing up or ironing, focus fully on the task in hand.

- When you go outdoors, use all of your senses to take in the sights, sounds and smells around you as you walk.

9. Assert yourself

Some experts believe that pain is often the result of bottled-up emotions and claim that expressing your true feelings can help to bring about a recovery from chronic pain conditions such as fibromyalgia. Whether or not this is true, assertiveness skills might be useful if you often agree to do things that you don't really want to do, or feel you are not up to doing, just to keep the peace or to keep other people happy.

Being assertive empowers you to say what you want, feel and need, calmly and confidently, without being aggressive or hurting others. The following techniques will help you to express your emotions and remain in control of your life, doing things because you want to, rather than to please other people.

- Show that you take full responsibility for your thoughts, feelings and behaviour by using 'I' rather than 'we', 'you' or 'it'. Rather than saying 'You make me angry', try something like 'I feel angry when you...' This is less antagonising to the other person.

- When you can choose whether to do something or not, say 'won't' or 'am not' rather than 'can't' to show that you've made an active decision, rather than suggesting that something or someone has prevented you. Say 'have decided' instead of 'have to' and 'could' rather than 'should', to indicate that you have a choice. For example: 'I am not going out tonight', rather than 'I can't go out tonight', or 'I could go out tonight, but I have decided to stay in'.

- When you feel that your needs aren't being taken on board, say what you want calmly and clearly, repeating it until the other person shows they've heard and understood what you've said.

- When asking for help, identify and communicate exactly what it is you want. Choose positive, assertive words, as outlined above. For example: 'I would like you to help me tidy the kitchen. I'd really appreciate it if you could empty the dishwasher.'

- When refusing a request, speak calmly but firmly, giving the reason or reasons why, without apologising. Repeat if you need to. For example: 'I won't babysit for you tonight because I'm feeling really tired after being at work all day.'

- When you disagree with someone, say so using the word 'I'. Explain why you disagree, while acknowledging the other person's right to hold a different viewpoint. For example: 'I don't agree that the service in that restaurant is poor – our meal was only late last time we visited because it was very busy, but I can understand why you think that.'

10. Find support

Fibromyalgia can be an isolating condition that leaves many sufferers feeling that no one understands what they are going through. Making contact with fellow sufferers who are dealing with the same symptoms as you may help to overcome these feelings. The organisations listed below offer the opportunity to do just that; further information and contact details can be found in the Directory at the end of the book.

UK Fibromyalgia – a UK charity that provides an online forum for fibromyalgia sufferers as well as a directory of fibromyalgia support groups across the UK.

FibroAction – a UK charity that provides details of local fibromyalgia support groups.

Fibromyalgia Association UK (FMA UK) – a UK charity that runs a telephone helpline, support groups across the UK and an online support forum for fibromyalgia sufferers.

Fibromyalgia-Support.net – a website that provides details of fibromyalgia support groups across the UK and runs 'FibroLads', a support group in Rugby for male fibromyalgia sufferers or men who are the partners of fibromyalgia sufferers. The group founder welcomes contact from men wishing to set up a similar group elsewhere.

Fibromyalgia Support Northern Ireland – a charity that provides an online directory of partly affiliated support groups in Northern Ireland, as well as an online forum and a drop-in service in Belfast and Coleraine.

HealthUnlocked.com – a website that offers a huge range of online communities to join – including one for fibromyalgia sufferers.

Patient.co.uk – a website offering health information 'as provided by GPs and nurses to patients during consultations', as well as forums where you can read about others' experiences of medical conditions (including fibromyalgia), medications, treatments and services – and share your own.

Help is at hand

If you feel you can't deal with life's stresses on your own, don't be afraid to seek professional help. Your first port of call should be your doctor, as they should be able to offer advice and possibly refer you to a counsellor.

The International Stress Management Association UK (ISMA) offers further guidance on dealing with stress, including how to recognise when you are stressed and stress-busting tips. See the Directory at the end of the book for contact details.

11. Laugh more

Laughter is a great stress and pain reliever. A good belly laugh appears to reduce the stress hormones cortisol and adrenaline, and raise mood-boosting serotonin levels. People who see the funny side of life appear to have a reduced risk of the health problems associated with stress. It's also thought that chemicals released when we laugh, such as endorphins and encephalins, can help to ease pain. Research at the University of Bath and Bath Royal National Hospital for Rheumatic Diseases found that patients with chronic arthritis pain who were able to laugh noticed their pain lessened afterwards. So make time to watch your favourite comedies and comedians and be around people who make you laugh. Or visit www.laughlab.co.uk or www.ahajokes.com whenever you feel like a good giggle!

12. Get closer to nature

Researchers at Essex University say that ecotherapy (engaging with nature) offers both mental and physical health benefits. Whether through an active pursuit such as walking or gardening, or a passive one like admiring the view, being close to nature has been shown to reduce stress and ease muscular tension. Experts claim that the higher levels of negative ions near areas with running water, trees and mountains may play a part. Others suggest that the success of ecotherapy is down to 'biophilia' – the theory that we all have an inborn affinity with nature and that our 'disconnection' from it is the cause of stress and mental health problems. Studies in the Netherlands and Japan suggest that people living in or near green areas enjoy a longer and healthier life than those living in urban environments.

Remember to tailor your activity levels to suit how you are feeling. On a 'good' day, engaging with nature might mean going for a walk in the park, or doing a spot of light gardening; on a 'bad' day, it might mean spending half an hour sitting in the garden soaking up some sunshine.

13. Practise relaxation techniques

According to Edzard Ernst, formerly professor of complementary medicine at the Universities of Exeter and Plymouth, meditation, hypnotherapy and relaxation may help improve fibromyalgia by relaxing the body and reducing anxiety about experiencing pain. Examples of how to practise these techniques are listed below for you to try.

Meditate

Research at Harvard has shown that mindfulness meditation significantly reduces pain in fibromyalgia. Mindfulness meditation involves focusing on your breathing to help you concentrate on the here and now, and distract you from any discomfort you are feeling. It also encourages you to breathe slowly and deeply – some experts link breathing too quickly (over-breathing) with a range of health problems, including poor concentration, fatigue and disrupted sleep patterns.

Simple mindfulness meditation:

1. Close your eyes and focus on your breathing.

2. As you inhale slowly and deeply through your nose, expand your stomach and hold for a few seconds.

3. Exhale slowly, drawing in your stomach.

4. Whenever your attention is distracted by a passing thought, return to simply observing your breathing.

Pain-relieving colour visualisation:

1. Think of a colour that suggests wellness to you – for example, green or blue.

2. Now think of a colour that represents pain to you – for example, black or red.

3. Now follow the meditation steps outlined previously.

4. On each inhalation imagine you are breathing in your 'wellness colour' and it is filling your whole body.

5. On each exhalation imagine you are breathing out your 'pain colour' and as you do so, all of the pain is flowing out of your body.

Self-hypnosis

Self-hypnosis involves picturing yourself as you would like to be, e.g. energetic and pain-free, while you are in a relaxed state.

Using affirmations (also known as mantras) helps to reinforce the image. An affirmation is a positive statement that describes what you want to achieve or feel in the present tense, as if it is already happening, with the idea that your subconscious mind will accept it as a reality. Here are some examples of affirmations for boosting energy and reducing pain: 'My body feels light and full of energy'; 'My muscles are relaxed'.

1. Breathe in and out slowly and deeply, as in the previous two exercises.

2. Now imagine yourself as you would like to be e.g. fit and well and doing activities you enjoy such as dancing or walking.

3. Repeat your chosen affirmation on each out-breath.

Relax your muscles

When your muscles are hurting, your natural response is to tense them, which leads to more pain. Learning to relax your muscles can help to break the cycle of pain and tension. A common way of relaxing the muscles is to first tense them and then relax them. However, if you have fibromyalgia your muscles are likely to be tight and tense already. Below is a gentler form of muscle relaxation:

1. Breathe in and out slowly and deeply, as in the previous exercises.

2. Now consciously 'invite' each muscle in your body to relax, starting with those in your face and neck, then your neck and shoulders, followed by your arms, your back and your buttocks. Finally, allow the tension to flow from your legs, including your thighs and calves.

Complementary therapies

Complementary therapies, particularly aromatherapy and massage, can also help to relieve stress. Details of complementary therapies can be found in Chapter 9 – Try DIY Complementary Therapies.

Chapter 3

Exercise to Ease Pain

The pain and fatigue associated with fibromyalgia, and the fact that exercise often makes the pain worse, or even triggers a flare-up, means that many sufferers avoid taking exercise. Yet exercise has been shown to be of benefit. A scientific review in 2008 concluded that moderate aerobic exercise may improve well-being and physical functioning, while strength training may reduce pain, tender points and depression – and bring about a big overall improvement. Examples of suitable moderate aerobic exercise include walking, rebounding (see Action 15), swimming and yoga. Appropriate forms of strength training include lifting light weights, or using a resistance band; as the name suggests, it improves your muscle strength and can make everyday activities, such as climbing the stairs and carrying shopping, easier.

Experts believe that exercise is essential for keeping muscles strong and flexible, and helping you stay active in other areas of life. In fact, exercise and activity allow patients to have some control over fibromyalgia and the amount of pain they feel.

Physical activity is thought to help ease the pain and depression associated with fibromyalgia because it releases pain-relieving and mood-boosting endorphins. Exercise can also be a social occasion if you attend classes, which can improve emotional well-being. Being active also aids weight management and improves sleep quality.

However, it is important not to overdo things by pushing yourself too far. It is best to gradually increase the length of time spent exercising and, if possible, break it up into two or three sessions. For example, start by exercising for five minutes two or three times a day, then gradually increase this to ten minutes two or three times a day. Always listen to your body – rest after a bout of exercise and view any worsening of pain, stiffness or fatigue the next day as a sign that you have done too much. If this happens, allow your body to rest and recover for two or three days, before restarting your exercise regime at a more modest level. Be especially careful not to overdo things during a flare-up.

14. Walk more

Walking is a great way to exercise when you have fibromyalgia – you can fit it into everyday life and it's free! You can also tailor how far and how quickly you walk according to your energy, mobility and fitness levels. If you're normally inactive it's best to build up gradually, perhaps initially walking for ten minutes each day, increasing to 15 minutes and then 20 to 30 minutes daily. Easy ways to fit more walking into your daily routine include walking to the shops, instead of driving or using public transport. Alternatively, you could get off the bus one stop earlier, or park the car further away from your destination. At work you could fit in a short walk at lunchtime and take the stairs instead of the lift. Walking your dog, or a neighbour's, is another way of ensuring you walk more.

15. Try rebounding

Rebounding is a low-impact aerobic exercise that involves marching or bouncing on a small, circular trampoline known as a rebounder. Research shows that rebounding not only boosts fitness and mood, but also improves posture, balance and co-ordination. Below is a suggested rebounding routine:

1. Stand in the middle of your rebounder with your feet shoulder-width apart. Now march slowly for two minutes, swinging your right arm as you lift your right foot and vice versa.

2. Start bouncing gently, without lifting your feet, for two minutes.

3. Now start lifting your feet as you bounce. Do this for two minutes initially, gradually building up to six minutes.

Safe rebounding

Don't bounce on a full stomach, or when you're feeling physically tired or unwell.

Don't wear slippery shoes or socks. Bounce in your bare feet, or well-fitting trainers or plimsolls.

Position your rebounder away from furniture.

For more information go to www.rebound-uk.com.

16. Get in the swim

UK Fibromyalgia recommends non-weight-bearing exercises, such as swimming in warm water, for sufferers who find that any kind of pounding exercise makes their pain worse. Recent research suggests that swimming can significantly reduce chronic pain in fibromyalgia; in a study involving 33 women with fibromyalgia, one group swam in warm water at least three times a week for one hour, while the other group didn't swim at all. At the end of the eight-month-long study, the women who swam reported a noticeable decrease in their pain levels compared with those who didn't.

There are a number of reasons why swimming can be helpful for people with fibromyalgia. When you are swimming the water supports your weight, which means it doesn't put much strain on your muscles and it helps to improve your mobility. It both strengthens and stretches the muscles and improves cardiovascular fitness. Warm water relaxes the muscles, helping to ease pain and stiffness.

Also, when you are swimming you have to focus on your breathing, rhythm and stroke, which takes your mind off your worries and encourages you to live in the moment. Swimming in the sea is especially relaxing, because it is another form of 'green exercise'. When you visit your local public swimming baths, if possible pick times when it isn't too busy, such as during weekdays or perhaps weekend evenings, to avoid being jostled or interrupted.

For information about swimming lessons visit www.swimtime.org. To improve your swimming technique visit www.swimfit.com, a website that offers animated swimming-stroke guides.

17. Say 'yes' to yoga

The word 'yoga' comes from the Sanskrit word 'yuj' meaning union. Yoga asanas (postures) and pranayama (breathing exercises) are aimed at uniting the body, mind and soul, and can be helpful in preventing and relieving fibromyalgia symptoms such as pain, 'fibro-fog', depression and sleep problems; hatha yoga is a slow, gentle form of exercise which not only strengthens the joints and muscles and improves posture, flexibility and mobility, but also relaxes tight, tender muscles, relieves stress and promotes calm. The word 'hatha' comes from the Sanskrit words 'ha', meaning sun, and 'tha', meaning moon, and means balance, which sums up the balancing effects the postures and breathing exercises have on the mind and body.

In 2010 researchers at Oregon Health and Science University in the US carried out a randomised controlled pilot study, involving 53 women diagnosed with fibromyalgia, to find out the effects of yoga on their symptoms and their ability to cope with their condition; 25 took part in eight weekly two-hour yoga sessions, while the other 28 received standard care. Those who practised yoga reported greater improvements in functioning, pain, energy, mood and ability to cope, compared with those who didn't.

Outlined below are a breathing exercise, two neck stretches and three asanas you may find beneficial:

Yogic breathing (pranayama)

Deep, yogic breathing has a calming effect because it counteracts the tendency to breathe too fast when you are stressed. It also promotes sound sleep.

1. Sit upright with your spine, neck and head aligned and your shoulders relaxed. Rest your hands, palms up, on your knees and close your eyes.

2. Inhale slowly and deeply, allowing first your tummy, then your chest to expand. Hold for a few seconds.

3. Now exhale slowly, pulling your tummy in. Hold for a few seconds. Repeat the sequence five times.

Sideways neck stretch

Take a deep breath in and, as you breathe out, slowly lower your left ear towards your left shoulder. Take another deep breath in and return your head to an upright position. Breathe out and lower your right ear towards your right shoulder. Repeat on each side three to five times. To increase the stretch, place the hand from the side you are stretching towards on the opposite side of your head and press gently.

Head to chest stretch

Take a long deep breath in, then breathe out slowly. Gently drop your head towards your chest, focusing on the stretch on the back of your neck. Slowly raise your head upright. Repeat three to five times.

The Tree (Vrksasana)

This asana calms the mind and improves concentration, helping to ease 'fibro-fog' and lift depression.

1. Stand up straight, with your feet slightly apart, and your neck, shoulders and arms relaxed.

2. Exhale as you place your left foot on the inside of your right thigh, as high up as you can, with your toes pointing downwards.

3. Inhale as you stretch your arms to your sides, with your fingers pointing downwards.

4. Exhale as you put your hands together in the prayer position.

5. Keeping your hands in the prayer position, raise your arms above your head. To keep your balance, concentrate on a point in front of you as you breathe in and out slowly and rhythmically. Hold the pose for about one minute.

6. Repeat on your other side.

The Cat (Bidalasana)

This asana, which mimics a cat stretching, relieves tension in the neck, shoulders and back, and encourages deep, calming breathing.

1. Kneel on all fours, with your head tilted backwards, and your arms and back straight. Your hands should be directly below your shoulders and your knees directly below your hips.

2. Inhale, allowing your tummy to expand as you hollow your back. Raise your head and look upwards. Hold for a few seconds.

3. Exhale, pulling your tummy in and arching your back as high as you can, curling your head inwards. Hold for a few seconds.

4. Repeat the sequence five times.

Half Spinal Twist (Ardha Matsyendrasana)

This asana will improve your spine's flexibility, relieve neck and shoulder stiffness, and boost your energy levels.

1. Sit upright on the floor with your legs stretched out in front of you.

2. Cross your right leg over your left leg, placing your right foot on the floor next to your left knee.

3. Grasp your right ankle with your right hand.

4. Place your left hand on the floor behind you, in line with your spine.

5. Turn your head and twist your trunk. Look over your left shoulder at your left hand.

6. Hold the posture, slowly inhaling and exhaling, rotating still further on each out-breath.

Learn yoga

The best and probably the most fun way to learn yoga is to attend classes run by a qualified teacher. To find one near you, visit the British Wheel of Yoga's website – www.bwy.org.uk. Or, if you'd prefer to learn at home, visit www.abc-of-yoga.com, a site that shows you how to achieve the various postures, using animated clips. You can buy CD and MP3 hatha yoga class downloads, suitable for all levels and abilities, and download a free 'taster session' at www.yoga2hear.co.uk. You can also find yoga information, products and guidance at www.yoga-abode.com.

Safe yoga

When practising yoga at home always proceed slowly and gently. Avoid forcing your body into asanas and stop if you feel any discomfort. Wear lightweight, loose clothing, to enable you to move freely and remove footwear, as yoga is best performed barefoot. Use a non-slip mat if the floor is slippery. Don't try inverted postures ('upside down' asanas, such as the shoulder stand) if you have a neck or back problem, or have high blood pressure, heart disease or circulatory problems. If in doubt, consult your GP first.

18. Strengthen your muscles

Strength training involves using resistance methods like free weights, weight machines, resistance bands or your own weight to build muscles and strength.

If you have mild to moderate fibromyalgia symptoms you may be able to safely use small weights of 225 g that wrap around your wrists or ankles and fasten with Velcro. You could start by using one and gradually build up to four. An easy way to use them is while you are walking around the house. Small dumbbells are also available. Before you begin any type of strength-training routine, it is advisable to get some guidance, perhaps from a physiotherapist, or an exercise coach or trainer at your local gym. They can give you advice on how many times a week and how long you should train, as well as what kinds of warm-up and cool-down exercises you should do before and after, to reduce the risk of worsening any pain or stiffness.

However, bear in mind that not everyone with fibromyalgia is able to do strength-training exercises, so always proceed carefully and stop if your pain worsens.

Chapter 4

Eat Foods that Fight Fibromyalgia

Research shows that fibromyalgia sufferers often have low levels of certain vitamins and minerals, and are more likely to be overweight or obese. A study published in *The Journal of Pain* in 2010 concluded that carrying excess weight makes pain sensitivity and sleep problems worse, and reduces physical strength and flexibility. The researchers also noted that weight loss often improves fibromyalgia symptoms. Research suggests that weight gain may be both a cause and effect of fibromyalgia; obesity has been linked to inflammation, which increases sensitivity to pain, and sufferers are often less active and prone to sleep problems, which are also linked to being overweight.

In this chapter we examine the role of diet in fibromyalgia and look at how eating a wholesome, balanced diet may prevent and relieve symptoms by keeping blood sugar levels steady, preventing weight gain and providing the nutrients your body needs for healthy functioning. The importance of ensuring you eat foods that supply antioxidants, B vitamins, vitamin D, various minerals and healthy fats, as well as those that boost 'good' bacteria in the gut, is discussed. We also explore how food intolerances can sometimes be involved in fibromyalgia. The benefits of drinking enough water, and avoiding too much caffeine and alcohol are explained. At the end of the chapter you will find a summary of the best foods to eat to help prevent and relieve fibromyalgia symptoms.

19. Balance your blood sugar

The brain needs a steady supply of glucose to function properly; low blood sugar is linked to fatigue, low mood, and poor memory and concentration – symptoms that many people with fibromyalgia suffer from. Choosing foods with a low glycaemic index (GI) is thought to be the best way to keep glucose levels steady and keep your energy, mood and brainpower on an even keel. These foods also help you to manage your weight because they keep you feeling full for longer.

The GI is a measure of how quickly a food raises the level of sugar (glucose) in the blood. Refined, starchy and sugary foods, such as white bread, cakes, biscuits and sweets, and sugary drinks such as pop, cola and squash, supply glucose in an easily absorbed form, which causes blood sugar levels to rise rapidly, only to fall just as quickly, leaving you craving more sugary foods and drinks. These foods and drinks usually have a high GI.

Complex carbohydrates found in wholegrains, such as porridge, wholemeal bread and brown rice, and fruit and vegetables such as apples, pears and oranges, sweet potatoes, carrots and sweetcorn, as well as pulses like beans and lentils, take longer to digest, so your blood sugar rises slowly and remains steady for longer. These foods tend to have a low GI. It is thought that the fibre content of these foods slows down the rate at which the body can absorb the glucose.

Bread containing wholegrains, such as granary bread, has a lower GI than wholemeal bread, because the grain has been ground in wholemeal bread, making it easier to digest.

The ripeness of a fruit and the cooking methods used also affect the GI. For example, a green, unripe banana has a lower GI than a ripe one, and boiled new potatoes have a lower GI than baked or mashed potatoes. Although fatty foods like chips, crisps and chocolate have lower GIs because their fat content slows down glucose absorption, they are best kept to a minimum because eating a lot of these foods will lead to weight gain.

Eating regularly also helps to stabilise blood glucose levels. Snacking on low-GI snacks in between meals, such as natural yogurt, oatcakes with cottage cheese or peanut butter (with no added sugar), berries, apples, oranges, or a handful of nuts or seeds, can help you avoid energy peaks and troughs.

20. Add some protein

Eating some protein alongside unrefined carbohydrates at each meal also helps to keep your blood sugar steady and boosts serotonin levels, too; protein slows down the rate at which glucose is released into the bloodstream and carbohydrate foods help the brain to absorb the tryptophan it contains. Tryptophan is an amino acid found in many protein-rich foods that the body uses to make serotonin, which is involved in the regulation of pain, mood and sleep; a lack of it is considered a causal factor in fibromyalgia. Protein-rich foods such as turkey, chicken, fish, eggs, meat, dairy foods, nuts, seeds, beans, lentils and wholegrains are particularly good sources of tryptophan. Other foods that supply tryptophan include bananas, avocados and dates.

21. Enjoy an ACE diet

Vitamins A, C and E are antioxidants. Antioxidants protect the brain and the body from damage from free radicals (oxidative stress) by neutralising them.

Free radicals are chemicals the body produces when it uses oxygen, and when it reacts to infection, stress, sunlight exposure and pollutants such as cigarette smoke, chemicals and food additives. They can damage the immune system, cause inflammation and lead to degenerative conditions; research suggests that oxidative stress may play a part in fibromyalgia; several studies have found that sufferers produce unusually high levels of a type of cytokine linked to inflammation. Cytokines are a type of white blood cell involved in the immune response.

There is evidence that people with fibromyalgia tend to lack these antioxidant vitamins and that eating more of the foods that supply them can be beneficial. In 2010 a Turkish study involving 30 fibromyalgia sufferers and 30 healthy volunteers concluded that people with fibromyalgia had lower levels of vitamins A and E. A 2001 study in the US involving 30 participants with fibromyalgia assessed the effect of an antioxidant-rich vegetarian diet that included raw fruits, salads and carrot juice over a period of seven months. The research concluded that 19 participants responded well to the dietary intervention and reported marked improvements in their fibromyalgia symptoms.

Vitamin A is also vital for tissue growth, and repairs and protects against respiratory infections. It comes in two forms – retinol and beta-carotene. Retinol is found in animal products such as liver, fish liver oils, egg yolks, whole milk, cheese and butter. Beta-carotene is found in plants – especially in yellow and orange fruits and vegetables such as carrots, sweet potatoes, butternut squash, cantaloupe melons, orange and yellow peppers, and apricots. Note: Excess retinol can be harmful, so don't take a fish liver oil supplement with a multivitamin. Pregnant women, in particular, need to be careful, as excess retinol can cause birth defects. Beta-carotene is not toxic.

> ### Tip: Roast vegetables in olive oil
>
> To help your body get more beta-carotene from vegetables like carrots, peppers and sweet potatoes, roast them in a healthy fat, such as olive oil. Roasting softens the cell walls, making the beta-carotene easier to digest. Adding fat helps the body to absorb it.

Vitamin C boosts immunity and is found in fruit and vegetables – especially citrus fruits, blackcurrants, berries, peppers (especially red), tomatoes, broccoli, potatoes, peas and cabbage. However, cooking these foods destroys some of the vitamin C they contain.

Vitamin E is found in nuts, seeds, avocados, sweet potatoes, olive oil and wheatgerm.

Note: There are many other antioxidants – eating a variety of different coloured fruits and vegetables helps to ensure that you obtain a wide range. For example, while the orange pigment in carrots, sweet potatoes and butternut squash supplies beta-carotene, another class of antioxidants called anthocyanins give fruits such as raspberries, strawberries, plums and blueberries their red, purple and blue hues, and lycopene is the antioxidant that gives tomatoes and peppers their orange and red colours.

22. Boost your B vitamins

Research suggests that many fibromyalgia sufferers have low levels of vitamin B1 (thiamine). A lack of this vitamin and vitamins B3 (niacin), B5 (pantothenic acid), B6 (pyridoxine), B9 (folic acid/folate), and B12 (cobalamin) can cause many of the symptoms associated with fibromyalgia, including fatigue, muscle weakness and pain, stiff joints, restless legs, sleeping difficulties, depression, irritability, poor memory, confusion and headaches.

B vitamins are also involved in energy release and the production of serotonin, so it is easy to see why ensuring you have an adequate intake of the B vitamins is important if you suffer from fibromyalgia.

A balanced diet containing meat, including liver and kidneys, fish, eggs, dairy foods, wholegrains, vegetables – especially green leafy vegetables and mushrooms – citrus fruits, beans, peas, nuts and seeds should supply enough B vitamins for most people's needs. If you're a vegan, or you eat a lot of processed foods, you may be lacking in B vitamins. Also, if you're stressed your body's requirements for these nutrients shoot up. In such situations you may benefit from taking a vitamin B complex supplement (see Chapter 5 – Benefit From Supplements).

23. Value vitamin D

Several studies suggest that a lack of vitamin D can be a contributing factor in fibromyalgia and other chronic pain conditions; a study by the American Society of Anesthesiologists in 2007, involving 267 chronic pain sufferers, concluded that one in four were short of vitamin D. Dr Michael Holick, a professor of medicine, physiology and biophysics at Boston University Medical Center, and a leading authority on vitamin D, believes that a lack of this vitamin is often misdiagnosed as fibromyalgia because the symptoms it causes are so similar; vitamin D deficiency is linked to muscle pain and weakness, bone pain and fractures, fatigue and depression, as well as sleep and digestion problems.

The recommended daily intake is between 10–15 mcg (400–600 international units) but nutritional therapists like Patrick Holford recommend at least double this amount – 30 mcg (1,200 international units) daily; two roll-mop herrings, or four canned pilchards, provide roughly this amount. For vegans, mushrooms are the only food source.

However, we get around 80 per cent of our vitamin D from the sun; the skin produces a form of it following exposure to sunlight. Many people in the UK are thought to be short of vitamin D because of a lack of sunshine – especially in winter when the sun's rays aren't strong enough. Exposing the skin on the face and arms to 30 minutes of sunlight daily (without sun cream) should provide enough vitamin D for most people. If you are fair-skinned and burn easily, limit your exposure to ten minutes, three times a day. Research in 2011 suggests that the safest time to sunbathe is before midday when the body produces higher levels of a protein that repairs skin damage from ultraviolet rays.

Vitamin D supplementation is recommended if you can't get outdoors, or if you don't eat good sources, such as oily fish, liver, eggs, milk and butter, or foods that are usually fortified with vitamin D, such as margarine, cereals and powdered milk. A standard serving of cod liver oil (15 ml/one tbsp) provides around 34 mcg (1,360 international units), but avoid taking a multivitamin tablet as well, as vitamin D is fat-soluble, which means any excess is stored in the liver and fatty tissues; high levels can be harmful (see Chapter 5 – Benefit From Supplements).

24. Mind your minerals

Magnesium

Magnesium has several crucial roles in the body. It is involved in the release of energy from foods and the production of serotonin, as well as healthy muscle function and the regulation of pain. It plays a part in the metabolism of the B vitamins and essential fatty acids, and has an important role in the absorption of calcium. Studies have suggested that many people with fibromyalgia have a low magnesium intake, which is not surprising, given that symptoms of a deficiency include fatigue, muscle pain, poor mental functioning, headaches, migraines, nervousness and insomnia.

Your magnesium levels may be low if you are stressed, or if you eat a lot of sugary foods. To ensure your intake of magnesium is adequate, eat plenty of nuts, seeds, dark green leafy vegetables (such as spinach, broccoli and kale), seafood, tomato puree, wholegrains (including cereals like All-Bran and Bran Flakes), oats, beans (including baked beans), peas, potatoes, bananas and yeast extract. Avoid drinking too much alcohol as it can hamper magnesium absorption (see Action 30 – Moderate your alcohol intake). Fizzy drinks are also best avoided, because the phosphates they contain also hinder magnesium absorption.

> ### Tip: Soak in an Epsom salt bath
>
> You can soak up magnesium through your skin by adding one or two cups of Epsom salts to the bath as it fills. The heat from the water also helps to soothe tender, aching muscles.

Calcium

Researchers have found that people with fibromyalgia are more likely to be short of calcium, which is needed for healthy muscles and strong bones; fibromyalgia primarily affects the muscles and is linked to reduced mobility, which can lead to osteoporosis (brittle bones) because bones need regular weight-bearing exercise to remain strong. Therefore it is sensible to ensure that your diet contains foods that supply this mineral. Women are more likely to suffer from osteoporosis after the menopause, when they lose the bone-protecting effects of oestrogen. Nutritionists recommend an intake of 1,000 mg a day, increasing to 1,500 mg daily for people aged 60 and over. Low-fat dairy foods, such as skimmed and semi-skimmed milk, yogurt, cottage cheese and reduced-fat hard cheeses, are the richest sources, because it is the watery part, not the creamy part, that supplies the calcium.

One pint (500 ml) of semi-skimmed milk, one 125 g pot of low-fat yogurt and 30 g of low-fat hard cheese supplies around 1,100 mg of calcium. Small fish, such as white bait and tinned sardines, pilchards, salmon and anchovies, are good sources – as long as you eat the bones. Good non-animal calcium-providers include almonds, Brazil nuts, seeds, tofu, soya, seaweed, figs, dates, dried apricots, purple broccoli, watercress, leeks, parsnips and dark green leafy vegetables such as kale, as well as lentils and beans.

To boost your absorption of the calcium they contain, sprinkle leafy green vegetables such as cabbage, broccoli, kale, and spinach, and salad greens, such as rocket, watercress and lettuce with a little ordinary vinegar or lemon juice. Drinking a tablespoon of cider vinegar in warm water, sweetened with honey if desired, once or twice a day is also recommended for promoting calcium absorption.

'Good' bacteria – probiotics such as lactobacillus – also seem to enhance calcium absorption (See Action 26 – Try probiotic power). Both calcium and magnesium have a tranquilising effect.

Chromium
Chromium helps to balance the blood sugar by working with insulin to remove excess glucose from the blood; we've already talked about how dips in blood sugar levels can lead to physical and mental symptoms such as fatigue, poor concentration and memory. Good sources of chromium include meat, wholegrains like oats and wholemeal bread, lentils, mushrooms and spices.

Zinc
The body uses zinc to make insulin, so it has an important role in maintaining blood sugar levels. It is also needed for a healthy immune system, and is involved in the production of neurotransmitters and growth hormone. A lack of zinc has been linked to abnormal pain responses, confusion and poor concentration.

Stress increases your requirements for zinc; the best sources are nuts, seeds, meat, eggs, seafood (mussels, prawns, sardines and oysters), beans, peas, mushrooms, broccoli, squash, spinach, kiwi and blackberries.

25. Have healthy fats

Fats have several important roles in the body, including ensuring the central nervous and immune systems work properly; a study published in the *International Journal of Clinical Pharmacology* in 2000 concluded that omega-3 fatty acids relieve muscle pain, improve mood and fight fatigue in fibromyalgia sufferers.

There are four main types of fat in the foods we eat:

- **Saturated** – mainly found in animal products, e.g. red meat, butter and full-fat dairy products. They are solid at room temperature and are thought to increase harmful low-density lipoproteins (LDL) cholesterol, increase inflammation and pain in the body, lead to atherosclerosis (hardening of the arteries) and make brain cells less flexible. They are also thought to make it more difficult for the brain to use polyunsaturated fats.

- **Trans (partially hydrogenated)** – found in some margarines and processed foods, such as biscuits, pies and cakes. These are made through a process called hydrogenation, which turns liquid vegetable oils into solid fats. If the EFA (see below) intake is low and trans fats intake is high, trans fats may replace EFAs in the brain, with detrimental effects on the way it functions. Trans fats may also cause blood-sugar disorders because they hamper the action of insulin.

- **Polyunsaturated** – essential fatty acids (EFAs), found in fish, vegetable oils, nuts and seeds, play a vital part in healthy brain function. The body breaks down the fats and oils we eat into fatty acids and can make some fatty acids from other substances, but it can't make polyunsaturated fatty acids, so we have to get them from food – hence they are known as essential fatty acids (EFAs).

There are two main types of EFAs: omega-3, found in oily fish, nuts, seeds, and some plant seed oils, such as flaxseed oil and rapeseed oil; and omega-6, mainly found in plant seed oils such as sunflower oil, corn oil and sesame oil, as well as meat. Both omega-3 and omega-6 fatty acids are needed for the brain and nervous system to function properly. Omega-3 oils are anti-inflammatory.

Monounsaturated (omega-9) – found in olive oil, rapeseed oil, avocados, nuts and seeds. These lower LDL cholesterol, are anti-inflammatory and also have a role in brain function.

Get the balance right

Getting the right balance between the two types of EFAs is important. Too much omega-6 can hamper the body's ability to break down omega-3 fats and, along with stress, can trigger inflammation, which hampers the body's ability to make serotonin from tryptophan; as we have already noted, low serotonin levels are linked to fibromyalgia and in particular to pain, fatigue, low mood, poor sleep, migraines and IBS.

UK diets are often too high in omega-6 fats, because many processed foods, cooking oils and margarines contain corn oil and sunflower oil – a ratio of omega-3 to omega-6 of around 1:10 instead of 1:3. So, to counteract inflammation, you should aim to eat more foods containing omega-3 oils and fewer containing omega-6 oils. There are two types of omega-3 fatty acids:

◖ **Long chain** – such as eicosapentaenoic acid (EPA) or docosahexaenoic acid (DHA) – found in oily fish, especially mackerel, herring, sardines, pilchards, salmon and fresh (not tinned) tuna.

◖ **Short chain** – for example, alpha-linoleic acid (ALA) – found in flaxseed oil, rapeseed oil, pumpkin seeds, sunflower seeds, almonds, walnuts, wholegrains, wheatgerm and soya beans.

Note: If your intake of these foods is low, experts recommend choosing a supplement containing at least 500–600 mg of EPA/DHA.

How much fat should I eat?

The current recommendation is that fats and oils provide no more than a third of your daily calorie intake. This is equal to around 70 g (5 tbsp) for women, of which no more than 20 g (1.5 tbsp) should be saturated fat, and 95 g (7 tbsp) for men, of which no more than 30 g (2 tbsp) should be saturated fats. To give you an idea of your daily intake, below is the approximate saturated fat content of an average portion of some everyday meals:

◖ Cheese and pickle sandwich: 10 g

◖ Fish and chips: 5.2 g (cooked in vegetable oil) or 22.7 g (fried in dripping)

◖ Sunday roast dinner: 9–14 g

◖ Lasagne: 12 g

◖ Curry: 20 g

◯ Pizza (per slice) – pepperoni: 9 g; seafood: 3 g; vegetable: 5 g

◯ Cheese omelette (made with two large eggs and 60 g of full-fat hard cheese): 18 g

To eat fewer 'bad' and more 'good' fats:

◯ Select lean meat and trim off visible fat. Remove the skin from roast chicken.

◯ Grill, bake, poach, steam, stew, pressure cook or microwave, instead of frying or roasting.

◯ Spoon off any fat that rises to the top when cooking stews or mince.

◯ Use more vegetables and less meat in stews and casseroles.

◯ Serve a high-fat food, such as meat pie or pizza, with a low-fat food, e.g. steamed vegetables or salad, for a more balanced meal.

◯ Opt for ready-meals with a lower fat content – check the label. Three per cent fat = low fat; 20 per cent fat = high fat.

◯ Measure oil when cooking – don't guess.

◯ When baking cakes, swap half the fat for low-fat yogurt.

◯ Use a low-fat spread, preferably containing olive or rapeseed oil, rather than butter or full-fat margarine.

- Avoid products with hydrogenated fat, hydrogenated vegetable oil, partially hydrogenated vegetable fat/oil or trans fatty acids listed in the ingredients.

- Choose low-fat yogurts, reduced-fat cheeses and semi-skimmed or skimmed milk.

- Grate cheese, so you use less.

- Avoid products with animal/saturated fats, shortening, glycerides, palm oils and milk fats in the ingredients list.

- Eat at least two portions of oily fish a week; it doesn't have to be salmon – tinned sardines on wholemeal toast is a cheap, nutritious meal that is rich in omega-3 fats.

- Eat up to 30 g (2 tbsp) of nuts and 15 g (1 tbsp) of seeds daily.

- Sprinkle seeds and chopped nuts onto your breakfast cereal and salads; add seeds to sandwich fillings; eat seeded breads and crispbreads.

- Use flaxseed, rapeseed or olive oil as a salad dressing and in cooking.

- Mash potato with olive oil, rather than milk and butter.

- Replace high-fat sauces and mayonnaises with balsamic or white wine vinegar, or strong condiments such as mustard and soy sauce, or herbs like basil, mint or coriander.

> **Spice it up**
>
> Use garlic and spices – especially cumin, ginger and turmeric – in your cooking, as there is evidence they ease pain and inflammation.

26. Try probiotic power

If you suffer from IBS or food sensitivity (intolerance) you might find including probiotics in your diet helpful. Probiotics are 'good' bacteria such as lactobacillus and bifidobacteria, which play an important role in digestion by helping to break food down further, and making important minerals like magnesium and calcium easier to absorb. They also prevent the more harmful strains of bacteria from multiplying by using up all of the available oxygen and nutrients.

Problems arise when levels of 'good' bacteria are reduced – perhaps after a bout of gastroenteritis or following a course of antibiotics, which destroy all types of bacteria. With fewer good bacteria present, the harmful strains, known as pathogens, can multiply. Research suggests that many IBS sufferers have lower levels of 'good' bacteria and higher levels of 'bad' bacteria such as E. coli and clostridium in the gut, which give off excessive amounts of gases and toxic waste products when they ferment food residues in the bowel, causing wind, bloating, pain and diarrhoea. This process is known as malfermentation and some researchers have suggested it could be a cause of food intolerances (see Action 27 – Check for food intolerances). Boosting levels of 'good' bacteria in your gut may help you control IBS symptoms; five randomised controlled trials (RCTs) showed that probiotics are good for reducing wind and bloating. Probiotics are also thought to boost immune function, which may be weakened when you suffer from fibromyalgia.

Terms used when referring to clinical trials

Double blind – a trial where information that might influence the behaviour of the investigators or the participants is withheld, e.g. which participants have been given a placebo, rather than an active substance.

Placebo – an inactive substance given to study participants to compare its effects against those of a treatment.

Placebo effect – a situation in which people taking a placebo feel better because they believe they have received a treatment and therefore expect to feel better.

Randomised controlled trials (RCTs) – viewed as the most reliable type of research trial because participants are randomly placed in a treatment group or a control group. The treatment group receives the treatment under scrutiny, while the control group receives a placebo or another treatment, for comparison. RCTs can be single blind, where the participant doesn't know which treatment they are receiving, or double blind, where neither the participants nor the researchers know who is receiving which treatment.

According to the World Health Organisation (WHO), probiotics are: 'Live microorganisms which, when administered in adequate amounts, confer a health benefit on the host.' WHO stipulates that for foods to be described as probiotic they should contain enough 'good' bacteria that are alive and active until the end of their use-by date, and can survive strong stomach acids. The label should state the type and strain of probiotic bacteria they contain.

Lactobacillus, bifidobacteria and streptococcus thermophilus types seem to be the most beneficial. Yogurt drinks such as Yakult and Actimel contain strains of lactobacillus and other probiotics, but these drinks can be high in sugar and some contain fructose as well, so choose 'light' versions where possible. You can also buy probiotic supplements, which usually provide high doses of probiotics, meaning more are likely to survive the acids in the stomach. Experts recommend taking a supplement containing lactobacillus and bifidobacterium with at least 10 million bacteria per dose. However, some of these can be expensive. Bio-yogurts are a decent source, too – although fruit yogurts tend to contain sugar or sweeteners, so natural yogurt is a healthier choice. You will probably need to take probiotics every day for at least a month before you notice any benefits.

> **You should cocoa!**
>
> Eating a little dark chocolate every day could help to boost your energy levels and mood; a small RCT at Hull York Medical School in 2007, involving ten people with chronic fatigue syndrome, found that those who ate 45 g of dark chocolate with 85 per cent cocoa content on a daily basis experienced less fatigue, depression and anxiety. The researchers concluded that the results were probably due to the high levels of polyphenols in chocolate boosting serotonin levels. The high magnesium content of dark chocolate might also have been beneficial.

27. Check for food intolerances

Some research suggests that food intolerances may play a part in some fibromyalgia sufferers' symptoms. In 2007 the medical charity Allergy UK conducted a survey of 5,200 people, of whom 59 per cent believed they had a food intolerance and 41 per cent thought they had a food allergy; 6 per cent of those surveyed said they suffered from aches and pains, 12 per cent said they experienced lethargy and anxiety, and 66 per cent reported interrupted sleep, as a result of their food sensitivities.

What is the difference between food allergy and food intolerance?

Food allergy, also known as immediate sensitivity, is where the immune system recognises a particular food as a foreign body and produces antibodies called immunoglobulin E (IgE) to fight it. This in turn leads to the body releasing chemicals such as histamine, which causes the allergic symptoms. Food intolerance, also known as delayed sensitivity or non-allergic hypersensitivity, isn't a true allergy, as it doesn't involve the immune response; see below for further information on identifying symptoms of a food intolerance.

How common are food allergies and intolerances?

Allergy UK says that food allergy is uncommon and only affects around two per cent of the UK population, whereas food intolerance is much more common, with up to 45 per cent of the UK population suffering from it. Some people suffer from both immediate and delayed food sensitivity.

However, not everyone accepts these figures; in 2010 researchers at Portsmouth University argued that only one in ten people in the UK who believe they have a food allergy or intolerance actually have one. They warned that self-misdiagnosis could mean people cut out certain foods unnecessarily, risking nutritional deficiencies, and advised anyone who believed they had food-related symptoms to visit their GP.

Food allergy

Food allergy causes symptoms within anything from a few seconds to up to three hours of eating the offending food. The symptoms are usually classic signs of allergy such as rashes, wheezing, itching, severe abdominal pain, nausea and vomiting. When the reaction is severe, it's known as anaphylaxis. Here, the symptoms are much more pronounced – there may be swelling of the lips, mouth and tongue. In extreme cases, there may be a sudden drop in blood pressure and loss of consciousness – anaphylactic shock – that in extreme cases can lead to death. Some researchers believe people who react in this way to certain foods may have a leaky gut wall. This is where it becomes over-permeable, perhaps as a result of stress, or irritants such as coffee, alcohol or some medications. In this state it allows partially digested molecules of food to enter the bloodstream, where they trigger a response from the immune system. Always call an ambulance immediately if you suspect an anaphylactic reaction.

If you develop a food allergy you are likely to become aware of it fairly quickly because of the rapid onset of symptoms that always happen in response to eating a particular food. Your GP may want to confirm precisely which foods you are allergic to by arranging for you to have a skin-prick test or a blood test to measure levels of IgE antibodies to particular allergens.

Food intolerance

In food intolerance the symptoms appear within four to 48 hours of eating the trigger food, hence it can be difficult to identify the culprit. A food intolerance is not life-threatening, but it can give rise to many of the symptoms associated with fibromyalgia, such as aches and pains, tiredness, bloating, nausea, diarrhoea, IBS, vomiting, headaches, migraine and sleep disturbances. It therefore seems probable that food intolerances are more likely to be involved in fibromyalgia than food allergies.

Food intolerances can be due to low levels of certain digestive enzymes, such as lactase, which breaks down milk sugars (lactose). Or they can result from a raised sensitivity to natural substances found in foods, such as salicylates (aspirin-like substances found in fruit, vegetables and other foods), caffeine and histamine found in foods like strawberries, cheese and chocolate. Food intolerance can be linked to commonly eaten foods such as wheat, dairy products, citrus fruits, eggs, beef, sugar and caffeine. Another possible cause is food additives – especially the artificial colouring tartrazine, the sweetener aspartame and the food flavouring monosodium glutamate (MSG). Aspartame and MSG in particular have been linked with fibromyalgia symptoms. Nitrates may also be a factor in some fibromyalgia sufferers' symptoms.

The aspartame and monosodium glutamate link

Aspartame is an artificial sweetener around 200 times sweeter than sugar, so the amount needed to give a sweet taste is so small it provides virtually no calories – hence it is used in diet drinks, yogurts and desserts. It is commonly found in low-sugar, sugar-free and diet foods and is usually listed on food labels under its original trade name NutraSweet, aspartame or E951.

MSG is a flavour enhancer that is often added to processed foods such as tinned soups, sausages and ready meals. It can be listed as E621 and is also present in other additives such as autolysed yeast, hydrolysed yeast, yeast extract, sodium caseinate, calcium caseinate, natural flavouring, vegetable protein, hydrolysed protein, gelatine and 'other spices'.

A small study published in *The Annals of Pharmacotherapy* in 2001 reported that when four fibromyalgia sufferers eliminated both monosodium glutamate and aspartame from their diets their symptoms were completely or greatly relieved. The research suggested that the findings could be due to both additives containing excitotoxins. Excitotoxins are substances that can stimulate the nervous system, particularly pain receptors, and therefore exacerbate pain. The research also claimed that when both aspartame and MSG are both present in the diet they may cause damage to the nervous system. It concluded that some fibromyalgia sufferers' symptoms may be due to sensitivity to aspartame and MSG. It might, therefore, be worthwhile cutting out foods and drinks containing these substances for a month or so to see if your symptoms improve (see below).

Keep a food diary

For many fibromyalgia sufferers, appropriate exercise, pacing, rest and relaxation, combined with a balanced diet and stress management, will lead to a marked improvement in their symptoms. However, if your fibromyalgia persists, it may be worth keeping a food diary to determine whether there is a link between what you eat and your symptoms. An ordinary notebook will do – simply jot down every food you eat and any symptoms you experience, such as pain, tenderness, stiffness, sleep disturbance, migraines, etc. daily for four to six weeks.

Sample food diary

Date	Time	Type of food eaten	Symptoms experienced	Time and duration of symptoms

If you notice a pattern emerging that suggests your symptoms could be linked to food intolerance, your next step should be to visit your GP, armed with this information. If your GP suspects food intolerance they may refer you to a dietician, who may advise following an 'exclusion and challenge test'.

Exclusion and challenge test

This involves avoiding eating the suspect food/foods for two to six weeks to see if your fibromyalgia symptoms improve ('exclusion'). You'll then be asked to reintroduce the food/foods one by one ('challenge') to see if your symptoms worsen again. Finally, you'll be asked to exclude the suspected foods again to see if your symptoms improve once more. Always follow this process under the supervision of your GP and a dietician to make sure that you follow a balanced diet throughout, as cutting out whole food groups can result in nutritional deficiencies.

> Select Food (www.selectfood.co.uk) is an online directory of companies that sell foods for people with allergies, such as wheat-free and dairy-free. For further details, see the Directory.

28. Drink enough water

Water is an important nutrient – your whole body, including your brain, needs sufficient water to function properly; it is involved in many processes within the body, such as the absorption of nutrients and the removal of waste. Research shows that drinking plenty of water boosts concentration and prevents symptoms of dehydration, such as headaches and fatigue – hence it is of obvious importance that people with fibromyalgia drink enough. Experts recommend 1.5–2.5 litres of water daily; this may sound like a lot, but remember foods like fruit and vegetables have high water contents, and therefore contribute to your daily intake. Also, tea and coffee can be counted as part of your fluid intake (they still contribute fluid, despite having a slight diuretic effect); however, they contain caffeine, so it's advisable not to drink too much, or to drink decaffeinated versions instead.

29. Cut the caffeine

Many fibromyalgia sufferers might be tempted to drink a lot of coffee for a much-needed energy boost. Coffee contains the stimulant caffeine, as do tea, cola and chocolate. A moderate amount of caffeine can boost both your energy levels and mood, and improve your alertness and concentration – which is especially useful if you are suffering from 'fibro-fog'. However, as the stimulant effects wear off, your energy levels are likely to dip, and too much caffeine can make you jittery and anxious, and make it difficult to fall asleep at night. Caffeine can also be addictive, because once the effects wear off your body craves more to give you another boost.

So if you consume a lot of caffeinated drinks and foods, such as coffee, strong tea, cola and chocolate, you might want to consider cutting your intake. The caffeine content of tea and coffee varies quite widely, depending on where the plants they are derived from are grown, the brand, how much coffee/tea is used and how long it is left to brew. It's hard to say how much caffeine is too much, as sensitivity to it varies from one person to another; however, most experts advise a daily limit of no more than 300 mg.

Decaffeinated coffee or tea, coffee substitutes made from chicory or dandelion, herbal teas and redbush (rooibos) tea are good alternatives to regular coffee and tea. Aim to wean yourself off regular coffee and tea gradually to avoid withdrawal symptoms like headaches and anxiety.

Caffeine content of drinks/foods

Drink/food	Average caffeine content
Tea (mug)	75 mg
Instant coffee (mug)	100 mg
Filter coffee (mug)	140 mg
Cocoa (mug)	7 mg
50 g plain chocolate	50 mg
50 g milk chocolate	25 mg

Herbal teas

Handy tip:
Use a cafetière to make your herbal teas quickly and easily. Place the herbs in the cafetière and add boiling water; replace the lid and leave to brew for a couple of minutes; press down the plunger and pour.

30. Moderate your alcohol intake

Some fibromyalgia sufferers find that drinking alcohol makes their symptoms worse, while others find that moderate drinking does not affect their symptoms and may even slightly improve symptoms such as pain. This could be because alcohol helps them to relax.

However, over-consumption of alcohol depletes various vitamins and minerals, including those that are needed for a healthy nervous system, such as B vitamins, calcium, zinc and magnesium, and amino acids such as tryptophan. As we've already discussed, deficiencies in these nutrients have been linked to various fibromyalgia symptoms – so even if you find you are able to tolerate alcohol, aim to drink moderately.

> Small amounts of red wine in particular appear to be beneficial to general health because it contains antioxidants such as resveratrol and catechins.

Another problem with alcohol is that it can cause or exacerbate sleep problems and disrupt normal sleep patterns (see Action 39 – Adopt good sleeping habits), hence it can worsen symptoms – especially fatigue. Also, if you suffer from depression or anxiety you may be tempted to self-medicate with alcohol, which could initially make you feel better because it temporarily boosts serotonin levels; however, when the effects wear off, you may be left feeling jittery and anxious, because it also stimulates the release of the stress hormone adrenaline and has a depressant effect that can exacerbate a low mood. Alcohol can also interact with some of the medications commonly prescribed for fibromyalgia, including anti-inflammatories, painkillers, antidepressants and sleep medications; always read the label, or speak to your GP or pharmacist, before drinking alcohol if you are taking any of these drugs.

Recommended safe alcohol limits:

Women: daily: 2–3 units; weekly: 14 units
Men: daily: 3–4 units; weekly: 21 units
One unit roughly equals: One small (125 ml) glass of wine; half a pint (250 ml) of beer or lager; one small glass of sherry or port; one single measure of spirits.
Note: Drinkers should also have at least two alcohol-free days each week to give the liver a chance to rest and repair.

Some tips to help you cut your alcohol intake:

- Alternate an alcoholic drink with a non-alcoholic drink.

- Drink a wine spritzer, which is wine mixed with soda, instead of just wine.

- Drink from a smaller glass.

- Buy smaller bottles of beer and lager.

- To learn more visit www.drinkaware.co.uk.

The fight-fibromyalgia diet

Below is a brief summary of the dietary advice in this chapter:

- Eat wholegrains and low-fat protein foods at every meal.

- Eat a variety of brightly coloured fresh fruit and vegetables.

- Eat oily fish at least twice a week.

- Use olive oil, rapeseed oil, flaxseed oil or walnut oil for cooking and on salads.

- Avoid processed foods high in saturated fats and additives.

- Use garlic, cumin, ginger and turmeric when cooking.

- Have bio-yogurts and probiotic drinks.

- Check for signs of food intolerance.

- Drink plenty of water.

- Moderate your caffeine and alcohol intake.

Chapter 5

Benefit from Supplements

This chapter looks at the various herbal, vitamin and mineral supplements that may help to relieve the symptoms of fibromyalgia, outlining what each supplement is, what it does, how it works and some of the evidence that it works, as well as advice regarding its safe use.

If you find it difficult to eat a balanced diet for whatever reason, supplements can help you to avoid nutritional deficiencies. They are controversial, with some researchers claiming that isolated substances don't provide the same health benefits as nutrients found naturally in foods. However, for many of us, supplements offer a convenient way to improve our diets and benefit from the specific properties of particular herbs, vitamins and minerals.

Do supplements work?

Often there is anecdotal evidence, but no, or insufficient, conclusive evidence that a supplement works. While there is a need to be cautious about unsupported claims, sometimes the lack of evidence is simply due to the fact that the research hasn't been done; even though the turnover in the herbal medicine sector is quite high, many individual manufacturers are unable to meet the high financial costs of clinical trials. So a lack of evidence to back up the use of a supplement doesn't necessarily mean it doesn't work, or isn't safe – but it is important to exercise some caution and make sure you only buy products from reputable companies. It is reassuring to know that the Medicines and Healthcare products Regulatory Agency (MHRA) has recently tightened up the regulation of herbal medicines and supplements to help ensure their effectiveness, safety and quality (see below).

Another problem is that some herbal remedies have several active ingredients, and this can make it difficult to identify which produce the beneficial effects. The quality of herbal medicines can also vary quite a lot due to differences in plant species, the type of soil they are grown in and methods of extraction and storage, etc. These variations can sometimes make it difficult to draw any firm conclusions about particular herbs.

Are supplements safe to use?

It is important to bear in mind that just because something is termed 'natural' it is not necessarily harmless. Vitamins, minerals and herbs contain chemicals that have an effect on the body, just as drugs do.

Supplements come under two categories: herbal medicines and food supplements, and are subject to legislation to help ensure the safety of those who use them.

Regulation of herbal medicines

According to the MHRA, a herbal medicine is any medicinal product that contains one or more herbal substances as active ingredients, or one or more herbal preparations, or a combination of the two.

Since the introduction of new legislation in April 2011, all herbal medicines must be registered under the Traditional Herbal Medicines Registration Scheme or hold a product licence. Registered herbal medicines have to meet specific safety and quality standards and carry agreed indications for when they should be used. Licensed herbal medicines have to meet specific standards of safety, quality and effectiveness. For more information go to: www.mhra.gov.uk/howweregulate/medicines/herbalmedicines.

Find out more

The MHRA provides a list of herbal products currently registered under the Traditional Herbal Medicines Registration Scheme, along with information sheets on their safe use. You can also report any adverse reactions from herbal remedies or supplements to the agency. Its contact details can be found in the Directory at the end of this book.

Regulation of food supplements

Vitamin and mineral supplements are defined as food supplements and come under the EU Food Supplement Directive. This legislation aims to protect consumers from unsafe products by ensuring all supplements are labelled correctly and only contain permitted amounts of approved vitamins and minerals. Manufacturers aren't allowed to make therapeutic claims about their vitamin and mineral supplements, i.e. they cannot say a herb or vitamin is a 'cure' for a particular ailment.

31. Take supplements

Vitamin B complex

What it is: Vitamin B complex is a group of vitamins that are found in a wide range of foods including meat, fish, dairy products, vegetables and wholegrains. You may be short of B vitamins if you eat a lot of processed foods, if you are a vegan or if you are under a lot of stress. Research suggests that many fibromyalgia sufferers are low in vitamin B1 (thiamine).

What it does: May help to relieve muscle fatigue and pain, depression and insomnia.

How it works: B complex vitamins are needed for normal muscle function, energy release, a healthy nervous system and for the production of serotonin. Fibromyalgia symptoms have been linked with high levels of homocysteine, an amino acid produced in the body. Supplementing with vitamin B complex has been shown to lower homocysteine levels.

Evidence it works: A 1997 study at the Institute of Neuroscience and Physiology at the University of Gothenburg, Sweden, involving 12 women with fibromyalgia, found that they all had high homocysteine levels and low levels of vitamin B12 in their nervous systems. The researchers reported a link between high homocysteine levels and fatigue, and concluded that low levels of vitamin B12 contributed to high homocysteine levels. Note: Supplementing with vitamin B12 alone can affect absorption of other B vitamins, so it is best to take a vitamin B complex supplement.

Available as: Tablets such as Solgar Formula Vitamin B-Complex '100' Tablets and caplets such as Holland and Barrett Complete B Vitamin B-Complex.

Safety: Taking B vitamins is generally safe. However, you should take a supplement containing no more than 100 mg of vitamin B6 – higher doses can cause nerve damage. If you are pregnant or breastfeeding, or suffer from gout, diabetes or liver problems, or have had a stomach ulcer, speak to your GP or pharmacist before taking a vitamin B complex supplement.

Capsaicin gel
What it is: Capsaicin is extracted from chillis.
What it does: It eases tenderness associated with fibromyalgia.
How it works: It reduces the levels of a protein called substance P, which is involved in the transmission of pain signals from the nerve endings to the brain, and in inflammation of the joints.
Evidence it works: An RCT looked at the effects of capsaicin gel on fibromyalgia. Forty-five participants were given either 0.25 per cent capsaicin gel four times a day, or a placebo gel, to apply to painful areas. After a month, those using the capsaicin cream had less tenderness and had much better grip strength than those using the placebo.
Available as: Capsaicin gel is available on prescription in the UK as a gel or a cream.
Safety: Capsaicin is an irritant, so keep the gel away from your eyes, nose, mouth and open wounds. Always wash your hands thoroughly after applying.

5-Hydroxytryptophan (5-HTP)
What it is: The body uses 5-HTP to make serotonin. 5-HTP supplements are usually made from the seeds of the Griffonia plant from West Africa.
What it does: Eases pain, clears 'fibro-fog', boosts mood and promotes sleep.

How it works: Serotonin helps to regulate mood, pain and sleep. Research suggests that people with fibromyalgia have low levels of serotonin.

Evidence it works: In a study published in *Alternative Medicine Review*, research concluded that supplementation with 5-HTP may relieve fibromyalgia-related pain, stiffness, fatigue, depression, anxiety and insomnia. However, some studies report no benefit. More research is needed.

Available as: Capsules such as Holland and Barrett 5-HTP capsules 50 mg and tablets such as Happy Days 100 mg 5-HTP with zinc and B vitamins.

Safety: 5-HTP should not be taken with SSRI (selective serotonin reuptake inhibitor) antidepressants such as Prozac, with weight-control drugs, or if you are pregnant.

Magnesium

What it is: A mineral some fibromyalgia sufferers have been found to be deficient in. It is thought that chronic fatigue affects levels of growth hormone, which in turn affects magnesium levels. A shortage is thought to contribute to muscle pain and fatigue. The form of magnesium most beneficial for the muscles is magnesium malate, which contains malic acid; malic acid is found in tart fruits such as apples and oranges.

What it does: Boosts mood and energy levels, relaxes the muscles and eases muscle pain.

How it works: Magnesium is involved in the production of energy and mood-boosting serotonin, and is needed for healthy muscle and nerve function. Magnesium malate reduces lactic acid in the muscles, which is linked to muscle pain and tenderness.

Evidence it works: A 2002 review for the medical journal *Clinics in Family Practice* concluded that 200 mg of magnesium twice a day, combined with 1,200 mg of malic acid once a day, eases fatigue, pain and tenderness.

Available as: Capsules such as BioCare Magnesium Malate 90 vegicaps.

Safety: Use with caution if you suffer from IBS, as magnesium can worsen diarrhoea.

SAMe (s-adenosylmethionine)

What it is: SAMe is a chemical compound found naturally in the body, produced from methionine, an amino acid found in high-protein foods, and adenosine triphosphate (ATP), a substance involved in the production of energy in the body.

What it does: Reduces pain, tenderness, fatigue and depression.

How it works: It is used by the body to make serotonin, a neurotransmitter involved in mood and pain regulation.

Evidence it works: Three out of four RCTs investigating the role of SAMe in the treatment of fibromyalgia reported that SAMe was more effective than a placebo in reducing both the number of tender points and/or the degree of tenderness felt, as well as symptoms of depression.

Available as: Tablets such as SAMe 400 mg enteric-coated tablets by BIOVEA.

Safety: Occasional mild side effects include nausea, headache, dry mouth, upset stomach and restlessness. More severe side effects – usually in people with depression – include anxiety and mania. Note: SAMe can increase the risk of bleeding if taken with blood-thinning medications like aspirin, heparin and warfarin.

Eleuthero

What it is: Eleuthero is a plant that grows in southeastern Russia, northern China, Korea and Japan. The parts of the plant used are the root and rhizomes (underground stems). It is also known as Siberian ginseng or Devil's shrub.

What it does: Helps to beat fatigue and improves mental alertness.

How it works: The active ingredients include eleutherosides and complex sugars, which help the body to produce energy.

Evidence it works: A study published in *Psychological Medicine* in 2004 concluded that eleuthero both reduced fatigue and improved energy levels in people with chronic fatigue. A review published in *Phytotherapy Research* in 2005 claimed that adaptogens like eleuthero can reduce pain, boost energy and improve sleep in fibromyalgia sufferers.

Available as: Tablets such as Lifeplan Siberian Ginseng 600 mg, capsules such as HealthAid Sibergin 2500 and Solgar Siberian Ginseng Extract, and liquid such as HealthAid Siberian Ginseng Liquid 50 ml.

Safety: Can occasionally cause diarrhoea when first taken, so use with care if you suffer from IBS. Don't take close to bedtime, as it can cause insomnia.

St John's wort

What it is: A hedgerow plant with yellow flowers.

What it does: Has an antidepressant effect similar to those of SSRIs and MAOIs (monoamine oxidase inhibitors). It also helps to ease nerve pain and has antiviral properties.

How it works: St John's wort boosts levels of the brain chemical serotonin, low levels of which have been linked to fibromyalgia. The active ingredient, hypericin, is thought to keep the brain chemicals linked to positive mood, such as serotonin and noradrenaline, in the brain for longer. It does this by blocking the effects of an enzyme that destroys them. Serotonin and noradrenaline are involved in the regulation of pain.

Evidence it works: There is no specific research regarding the effects of St John's wort supplementation on fibromyalgia symptoms;

however, antidepressants with similar brain-chemical-boosting actions have been shown to help treat pain and depression associated with fibromyalgia.

Available as: Tablets such as Kira Good Mood St John's Wort Extract 450 mg and Nature's Best St John's Wort High Strength One-a-Day.

Safety: Warning: If you are taking any kind of medication, seek advice from your GP or pharmacist before taking St John's wort, as it can react with several commonly prescribed drugs, including the contraceptive pill, anti-epileptic drugs, warfarin and the antibiotic tetracycline. It can enhance the effects of SSRI antidepressants and should not be taken by anyone with bipolar disorder. It can also increase sensitivity to sunlight.

Red Montmorency cherries

What they are: A type of tart cherry grown in North America.

What they do: Help to maintain muscle strength, ease pain and improve sleep patterns.

How they work: The cherries are rich in antioxidants called anthocyanins and flavonoids which reduce inflammation. They are also rich in the 'sleep hormone' melatonin.

Evidence they work: In 2011 researchers at the Oregon Health & Science University reported that drinking tart cherry juice helped to maintain muscle strength and reduced overall pain. Another study in 2011, at the Northumbria Centre for Sleep Research at Northumbria University, found that volunteers who drank red cherry juice slept more soundly and for longer.

Available as: Juice such as CherryActive Concentrate, capsules such as CherryActive Capsules and dried cherries such as CherryActive Dried Montmorency Cherries.

Safety: There are no reported safety issues associated with taking this supplement.

Vitamin D

What it is: A fat-soluble vitamin often known as 'the sunshine vitamin' because it is produced in the skin following exposure to sunlight. It is also found in foods like oily fish, eggs and liver, as well as fortified cereals and margarine. If you don't eat these foods regularly and don't get outdoors much you could benefit from supplementation; recent research suggests that a lack of vitamin D can cause symptoms linked to fibromyalgia, including muscle pain, fatigue, low mood, and sleep and digestive problems.

What it does: Relieves muscle pain, boosts mood and promotes sound sleep.

How it works: Vitamin D improves absorption of calcium, low levels of which are associated with muscle and bone pain. Calcium is also needed for a healthy nervous system and calm disposition. Vitamin D is also involved in the production of serotonin, from which the body also makes the 'sleep hormone' melatonin.

Evidence it works: A study in the Middle East, published in *Clinical Rheumatology* in 2009, found that 90 per cent of patients diagnosed with fibromyalgia and/or musculoskeletal pain improved when treated with vitamin D supplements. Several studies suggest that vitamin D supplementation can improve mood, including a double-blind trial in which healthy people were either given 400–800 international units (IU) of vitamin D daily, or no vitamin D, for five days during the winter.

Available as: Caplets such as Holland and Barrett Sunvite Vitamin D3 25 mcg (1,000 IU), capsules such as Solgar Vitamin D3 Softgels 25 mcg (1,000 IU), and fish liver oil such as Seven Seas Pure Cod Liver Oil.

Safety: According to the US National Institutes of Health, the safe upper limit of vitamin D for people aged nine years and over is 100 mcg (4,000 IU) per day, but in general up to around 30 mcg (1,200 IU) should suffice. Fish liver oils such as cod liver oil supply vitamin A as well as vitamin D. The recommended daily amount (RDA) for vitamin A is 0.7 mg for women and 0.6 mg for men. Taking too much vitamin A can be dangerous, as any excess is stored in the liver. High levels can cause damage to the bones and liver, as well as double vision, vomiting, headaches and hair loss. Pregnant women should not take fish liver oils, as vitamin A can cause birth defects. If you eat liver regularly you should not take fish liver oil.

Check the benefits

To decide whether it is worth continuing to take a supplement, check the effects it is having on your fibromyalgia symptoms. Evaluate your symptoms on a scale of nought to ten before supplementation, then repeat after three months of use. Only try one supplement at a time, otherwise you won't know which one is beneficial. If you think a particular supplement is helping you could double check by stopping it for a short time to see if your symptoms worsen again.

Chapter 6

Live Better with Fibromyalgia

The pain and fatigue of fibromyalgia can make everyday activities difficult. This chapter offers practical advice to help you cope, including ways to manage a flare-up and to deal with household chores, driving, working and travelling.

32. Manage a flare-up

How can you cope with everyday life when you are suffering from a painful fibromyalgia flare-up? Below are a few tips to help you manage your next flare-up and, hopefully, reduce its impact.

☐ **Apply heat** – heat from a hot water bottle, a hot bath or shower, or a pad or wheat pillow that can be heated in the microwave (see Useful Products) helps to relax the muscles, thereby relieving pain and stiffness. For stiff, aching hands, fill the washbasin with warm water, apply a little oil (baby oil or vegetable/olive oil will do) and massage your hands underwater.

Have a massage – ask a partner or friend to give you a massage. This will help to ease sore muscles and lift your spirits (see Action 49 – Massage away pain).

Identify possible triggers – then do what you can to eliminate them. For example, if you suspect stress is to blame, try stepping back from difficult situations, or even arrange to take a short break if you can – see Chapter 2 – Pace Yourself, Rest and Relax.

Slot in more sleeping time – you could do this by going to bed earlier or having a lie-in. If you are having problems sleeping, follow the sleep hygiene advice in Action 39 – Adopt good sleeping habits, further on in this chapter.

Adjust your exercise levels – if you think you might have done too much physical activity lately, ease up a little. If you've let your exercise routine slide recently, try doing some gentle yoga stretches (see Action 17 – Say 'yes' to yoga).

Take your mind off the pain – by doing relaxing activities you enjoy. For example, focusing on reading, painting, knitting or sewing can prove to be a welcome distraction.

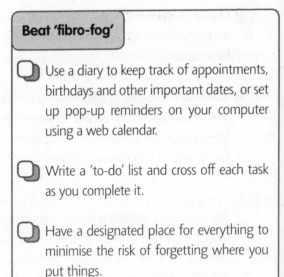

Beat 'fibro-fog'

☐ Use a diary to keep track of appointments, birthdays and other important dates, or set up pop-up reminders on your computer using a web calendar.

☐ Write a 'to-do' list and cross off each task as you complete it.

☐ Have a designated place for everything to minimise the risk of forgetting where you put things.

33. Keep on top of household chores

Keeping on top of household chores can seem nigh on impossible when you are struggling with fatigue and pain. Below are some tips to help you cope:

☐ Aim at cleaning one room at a time, rather than the whole house. If it is a big room break it down into small areas and have a rest in between tackling each one.

☐ On a bad day only clean the areas where high standards of hygiene are needed, e.g. the toilet and hand basin, the kitchen sink and worktops.

- Choose a lightweight vacuum cleaner – and if you live in a house, have one upstairs and one downstairs, so that you don't have to carry it far.

- Avoid clutter by putting things away after you've used them and encourage other people in the house to do the same. Throw away things you don't need, or don't use. For more tips see Action 6 – Clear away clutter.

- Delegate the chores you don't have the energy to do. Even children can help with tasks like emptying wastepaper bins or washing up.

- Keep a basket near the bottom of the stairs so that you can carry several items upstairs together instead of making more than one trip.

- Choose clothes made from easy-care fabrics that need little or no ironing.

- When you're feeling well cook extra portions and put them in the freezer in readiness for when you're not feeling so good.

- If you find it too painful to peel fresh vegetables keep a supply of frozen vegetables in the freezer – they are just as nutritious.

- Keep utensils you use a lot in easy-to-reach places.

Speedy clean

If you are expecting a visitor but don't have the time or energy to give the whole house a clean, focus on sprucing up the main areas your guest is likely to see instead, i.e. the living room and the toilet.

1. Whisk a feather duster or an absorbent cloth over the furniture, mantelpiece and windowsill.

2. Quickly sweep or vacuum the areas of the floor that need it.

3. Fluff up the pile on any rugs with your hand.

4. Plump up and straighten the cushions.

5. Light one or two scented candles, or an aromatherapy oil burner.

6. Clean the toilet.

34. Complete tasks more easily

When cooking vegetables in a pan, place them in a metal colander. When they are cooked, lift them out in the colander – this saves lifting heavy pans to drain them. Try filling the kettle using a lightweight plastic jug, using just enough water for your needs; and sit on a kitchen stool when preparing meals.

The following equipment might make housework easier:

- Long-handled sponges for washing up – but if you have stiff fingers, placing them in warm water may be therapeutic.

- Kitchen gadgets such as a rubber cap gripper, kitchen knives and vegetable peelers with padded handles, an electric tin opener and food processor.

- Lightweight mugs, pans and kettle, and plastic crockery, if you find the normal kind too heavy.

- Long-handled tools with a gripping mechanism, known as 'reachers', to retrieve items that are hard to reach; and a long stick with a rubber end for pushing the buttons on the television and microwave.

- A feather duster to dust hard-to-reach areas.

- 'Push-on' clothes pegs, rather than those with a spring mechanism.

- A lightweight, hand-held vacuum cleaner to clean upholstery and stairs.

- Fitted sheets that don't need to be tucked in.

- A trolley to move items from room to room.

Empty soap dispensers – if you find squeezing shampoo and conditioner bottles problematic, you can fill the dispensers with shampoo or conditioner, then label.

35. Clean naturally

In the introduction we mentioned how chemical sensitivity is a common fibromyalgia trigger. In a recent study by the World Wildlife Fund involving 47 volunteers, up to 54 man-made chemicals were detected in individual volunteers' bodies. Many of these were found to have come from household cleaning products and were identified as harmful. Some researchers believe that exposure to these and other chemicals may play a part in many people's fibromyalgia symptoms; so instead of using products laden with chemicals, opt for eco-friendly cleaners based on natural ingredients, such as Ecover or one of the supermarkets' own brands. Alternatively, you can make your own using items from your kitchen cupboard, such as bicarbonate of soda, lemons, vinegar and salt.

Soda solution
Bicarbonate of soda is cheap and very versatile. Mixed with water, it forms an alkaline solution that helps dissolve dirt and grease and neutralise smells.

Use a bicarbonate of soda solution on carpets to remove stains.

To remove odours from carpets sprinkle with dry bicarbonate of soda, leave for at least 15 minutes, then vacuum off.

To clean a smelly drain, sprinkle one cupful of bicarbonate of soda into it, then slowly pour one cup of white vinegar down. The resulting foam degreases and deodorises.

Sprinkle onto a damp cloth, and use as a mild abrasive to remove marks from plastic, porcelain, glass, tiles and stainless steel surfaces without scratching.

Fill a small container with bicarbonate of soda and leave in the fridge to absorb odours. Stir it now and again and replace every three months.

To clean and freshen your dishwasher add one cup of bicarbonate of soda and run it on the rinse cycle while empty.

For tough stains, mix with a little water to make a paste, apply and leave for a few minutes, before rinsing off. Silverware and jewellery emerge bright and shiny when cleaned in this way.

Lemon fresh

Lemons contain citric acid, which makes them great natural cleaners, with bleaching, antiseptic, antibacterial and degreasing properties.

Use half a lemon to clean the bath and washbasin. Rubbing it on and around the taps will remove limescale and leave them sparkling – especially if you buff them afterwards with a dry cloth.

To clean copper and brass, dip half a lemon into salt and rub. Rinse well straight away to prevent discolouration.

◯ Lemon is also a natural bleach – to brighten clothing and bed linen, soak them in a bucket of water to which you've added the juice of a lemon and leave overnight, before washing as normal.

◯ Lemon also deodorises. To clean your microwave and remove food smells, place a couple of slices of lemon into a microwaveable bowl containing water. Microwave for a couple of minutes, then wipe using kitchen roll or a clean cloth.

◯ To keep your fridge fresh, place a couple of slices of lemon inside.

Natural polish

Olive oil is a great natural substitute for commercial furniture polish. Simply mix a cup of ordinary olive oil – it doesn't need to be extra-virgin – with the juice of one lemon and pour it into a spray bottle. To polish wooden surfaces, spray a little on to the surface and rub. The lemon juice cuts through the dirt, while the olive oil shines and protects the wood. Use a dry cloth to remove the excess oil and buff to a shine. Use sparingly, as excessive amounts of oil could leave the surface feeling sticky. Olive oil is also good for getting rid of fingerprints on stainless-steel surfaces and cooking utensils. Simply sprinkle a little on some kitchen roll and buff.

Versatile vinegar

Vinegar is a dilute solution of acetic acid that cuts through grease, deodorises and disinfects. White vinegar is the best type to use around your home, as it doesn't have a strong smell. Mix equal amounts of white vinegar and water in a spray bottle, and use as a general cleaner. It's especially good on tiles and kitchen worktops, and for removing mildew. For a fresh fragrance add a few drops of lemongrass, bergamot or geranium essential oils. For difficult stains, use warm water; cover the stain and leave for ten minutes before wiping off. White vinegar also makes an excellent window cleaner – use half a cup in a litre of warm water. Simply spray onto your window and then remove and buff with crumpled newspapers to avoid streaking.

Vinegar is a good de-scaler, as it can dissolve lime deposits. To clean a showerhead, simply remove it and soak in undiluted vinegar. To remove limescale from your kettle, fill it up with vinegar and leave overnight. Pour the liquid out the next day and rinse well before using. To de-scale taps, soak a few paper towels in white vinegar. Wrap them around the taps and then cover them with plastic bags held in place with elastic bands. Leave for a few hours before rinsing and buffing to a shine with a dry cloth.

Ketchup cleaner

If you've run out of vinegar, tomato ketchup makes a good, if slightly messy substitute, as it contains acetic acid. It's especially recommended for cleaning copper and brass.

Aromatic air freshener

Instead of using commercial air fresheners to remove bad smells, try making your own. Fill a spray bottle with white vinegar and add about twenty drops of an essential oil of your choice, for example, lemon, geranium or peppermint. Shake well before spraying. Avoid spraying near your eyes, as vinegar can irritate them.

Natural disinfectant

Australian tea tree oil – *Melaleuca alternifolia* – is an excellent disinfectant and fungicide. For a general-purpose disinfectant solution, mix 10 ml (2 tsp) of tea tree oil with two cups of water. To remove and reduce mould and mildew growth, use the solution in a spray bottle and squirt on the affected areas. Leave for a few minutes and then rinse with warm, soapy water. To keep shower curtains mildew-free and to remove strong mildewy smells from fabrics, add a few drops of tea tree oil to your usual washing powder.

Bleach substitute

Borax (a natural mineral salt containing boron) can be used as a gentler alternative to bleach. To remove stains on white cotton or linen, apply directly, then rinse. Soak coloured fabrics in a weak solution of borax – made by adding 20 g (one tablespoon) to 500 ml (1 pint) of water – for no longer than 15 minutes. For an all-purpose household cleaner and disinfectant, mix one teaspoon of borax with two tablespoons of white vinegar and one litre (2 pints) of hot water.

36. Drive more comfortably

Fibromyalgia can affect every aspect of your life – including driving. Many fibromyalgia sufferers report having problems when they drive for any length of time, because it aggravates the pain. Below are some pointers that may help you to drive more easily and comfortably.

Perfect your posture

Posture is just as important when you are driving as any other time. Adjust your seat so that you are close to the steering wheel. This makes you less likely to slouch, or to strain to reach the pedals. Angle the seat at 100–110 degrees to encourage you to sit correctly.

Hold the steering wheel at 'quarter to three' position to help prevent arm, shoulder and back pain.

Pace yourself

Pacing yourself is just as important when driving, so make sure you take regular breaks. Whenever you take a break, get out of the car and go for a short walk, or do a few stretches. If you have to drive a long distance, consider completing the journey over two days, with an overnight stay in between, to ensure you don't overdo things, or share the driving with your partner or a friend.

Hot seat

If your car has heated seats, turning the heat on can help to soothe aches and pains. If you don't have heated seats you can buy car seat covers that heat up.

Ease the strain

If your hands are painful, use a wide car-key holder to make it easier to turn on the ignition. Wear thin driving gloves to make it easier to grip the wheel.

Cover the seat with a silk scarf to make it easier for you to twist around when you get in and out.

37. Adapt your work situation

Working with fibromyalgia can prove difficult – statistics suggest that up to 30 per cent of sufferers are forced to cut their working hours or to take on a less demanding job. Of course, this depends on the level of disability. However, employment not only improves your financial position, but can also boost your physical and emotional well-being.

The Disability Discrimination Act (DDA) states that employers must not discriminate against a disabled person in the workplace, and covers a range of issues including recruitment and the provision of appropriate facilities to enable you to do your job. Not everyone with fibromyalgia is covered by the DDA. According to the Act, a disabled person is someone with 'a physical or mental impairment which has a substantial and long-term adverse effect on their ability to carry out normal day-to-day activities'.

You would be covered if you have significant mobility problems, loss of function in one or both hands, chronic pain or difficulty lifting heavy objects, because of fibromyalgia. If the Act applies to you, you have the right to 'reasonable adjustments' to help you carry out your job. Even if you are not considered disabled, it is still good practice for your employer to adapt to your needs. These adaptations could include:

○ **Flexible working** – this might mean being able to start and finish work later, if your symptoms are usually worse in the mornings. You may be able to work from home, and also have time off for medical treatments and physiotherapy.

○ **Changes to your work environment** – this could include improving accessibility to your work area, providing special equipment or making adaptations to tools, adjusting work furniture or modifying your job role.

Reduce the strain at work

If your job involves spending long spells sitting at a desk, there are several steps you can take to reduce the levels of pain, stiffness and discomfort you experience.

○ Place the documents and files you use the most within easy reach.

Sit up straight to avoid unnecessary muscle strain – your ears, shoulders and hips should all be aligned.

Your shoulders should be relaxed, not hunched, and your hands, wrists and forearms should all be more or less parallel to the floor.

Adjust your chair so that your feet are flat on the floor. Your knees should be at the same level as, or slightly lower than, your hips.

Your keyboard should be at the same level as your elbows and your wrists should be horizontal when you are typing.

Your computer screen should be around 46–63 cm from your eyes and positioned so that you're looking straight ahead; the top of the screen should be in line with your eyes.

If you suffer from pain in your hands, ask for a wrist rest, an ergonomic keyboard and a trackball mouse, which is easier to operate and can reduce strain.

Keep the mouse close to your keyboard to lower the risk of shoulder and arm strain.

If finger stiffness makes typing difficult, ask for a keyboard guard – this makes it harder to hit the wrong key and also provides a platform on which you can rest your hands.

If you use a telephone frequently you could ask for a telephone with large push buttons and a hands-free headset.

Get up from your desk and walk around at least once an hour to prevent muscle stiffness.

If you are not sure whether your workspace is appropriate for your needs, ask your employer to check that it complies with health and safety regulations. An occupational therapist can advise you on suitable changes and devices to help you do your job.

38. Enjoy travelling

Going on holiday is a great way to relieve stress, with the added bonus that if your destination is in sunny climes the warmth can help to relax the muscles and ease pain.

If you have mobility problems let your travel operator know when you book, so that they can ensure your needs are met, e.g. that your resort, hotel and room are easy to access.

If your mobility problems are severe, consider using a specialist travel company that provides holidays tailored to your needs (see Useful Products).

Use lightweight luggage with wheels and pack as few items as you can, to avoid having to carry a heavy load.

Pack essential medications in your hand luggage.

Prepare for a possible flare-up while you're away – ensure you pack items you usually rely on to help you cope, e.g. a relaxation tape or your favourite massage oil.

Avoid overdoing things by allowing yourself plenty of time to reach the station or airport.

Travel mid-week when airports and stations are likely to be less crowded, which means queues will be shorter.

Reserve an aisle seat on a bus or plane to make it easier for you to get up and stretch your legs, and to do simple arm stretches to ease stiffness and pain.

Pop travel cushions or pillows in your hand luggage for extra support and comfort (see Useful Products).

Wear comfortable clothing. Layers are a good idea, as you never know when you are going to be too hot or too cold.

Allow for time differences when taking your medications.

Remember you need to pace yourself, even when you're on holiday; alternate spells of sightseeing with periods of rest.

Chapter 7

Cope with Other Fibromyalgia Symptoms

Poor sleep, migraines, irritable bowel syndrome (IBS), restless legs syndrome (RLS) and Raynaud's are all part of the fibromyalgia syndrome. Interestingly, fibromyalgia, insomnia, migraines, IBS, and Raynaud's have all been associated with imbalances in the neurotransmitter serotonin, while RLS is linked to low levels of dopamine, another neurotransmitter.

Often one symptom can trigger another, for example, fibromyalgia pain or RLS can cause insomnia, which can raise stress levels and trigger migraines and depression, as well as exacerbate other fibromyalgia symptoms.

In this chapter you will find an overview of the symptoms of each condition and effective ways to manage them.

39. Adopt good sleeping habits

A 2010 study at the National Research Centre for Stroke, Applied Neurosciences and Neurorehabilitation in Auckland, New Zealand, involving 16 fibromyalgia sufferers, found that poor sleep dominated their lives; the greatest difficulty they experienced was going back to sleep after waking up during the night. The study concluded that fibromyalgia sufferers should be screened for sleep problems and given advice on how to manage any sleep difficulties.

Research in 2011 at the Norwegian University of Science and Technology in Trondheim, Norway, concluded that the risk of developing fibromyalgia was five times higher among women aged over 45 who reported 'often' or 'always' having sleep problems. Other studies have also suggested a link between sleep problems and fibromyalgia, but it isn't clear whether sleep problems cause fibromyalgia, or fibromyalgia causes sleep problems. The pain and depression associated with fibromyalgia can cause difficulty sleeping, and lack of sleep can worsen depression, 'fibro-fog' and fatigue, leading to a vicious cycle of lack of sleep and worsening symptoms. Sleep problems can also be a side effect of certain medications taken for fibromyalgia-related depression and pain. Lack of sleep can also raise your risk of other health problems, such as obesity, high blood pressure and diabetes.

Whether sleep problems are a cause or an effect of fibromyalgia, if you don't sleep well it is clearly important that you take steps to improve your sleep. To sleep more soundly try these tips:

- **Take steps to ease any pain before bedtime** – this might involve applying a pain-relieving gel, or taking appropriate painkillers, taking some gentle exercise, or perhaps asking a partner or friend to gently massage the painful areas.

- **Keep your bedroom cool** – your brain tries to lower your body temperature at night to slow down your metabolism and encourage sleep. A temperature of 16–18°C is ideal.

Block out the light – use dark, heavy curtains; darkness stimulates the pineal gland in the brain to release melatonin.

Choose a mattress that gives you the correct support – if you lie on your back you should be able to slip a hand under your lower spine. If there's no gap, the mattress is too soft for you; a bed board under the mattress could help. If there's a lot of space, the mattress is too hard.

Pick a pillow that keeps your spine aligned with your neck – the best pillow thickness for you will depend on the width of your shoulders; if your shoulders are narrow choose a fairly flat pillow; if you have broad shoulders, you might need two pillows.

Banish TVs, computers, iPads and mobile phones from the bedroom – to help your brain associate your bedroom with sleep and sex only. Switch off your computer, mobile phone and other technology a couple of hours before bed to help you switch off.

Get outdoors in daylight – this stops the production of the 'sleep hormone' melatonin, making it easier for your body to release it at night. Blue light, which is light from a clear blue sky, is believed to be the most beneficial.

Eat tryptophan-rich foods – such as dairy products, chicken, turkey, bananas, dates, rice, oats, wholegrain breads and cereals. Tryptophan is an amino acid from which your body produces serotonin, which it uses to make melatonin.

Avoid drinking coffee or cola after 4 p.m. – the caffeine they contain can stimulate the brain for hours. While tea has between half to three-quarters as much caffeine (roughly 50 mg per cup and 75 mg per mug), if you are especially sensitive, avoid drinking it near bedtime. Redbush (rooibos) tea or herb teas, which are caffeine-free, make good alternatives.

Try a valerian supplement – also known as 'nature's valium', this traditional herbal remedy has been shown to promote relaxation and sleep.

Don't go to bed hungry or too full – both can promote wakefulness.

Exercise encourages sleep – because your body temperature and metabolism fall a few hours later. However, avoid exercising after 8 p.m. as your body temperature could still be raised at bedtime, promoting wakefulness. Insufficient exercise can cause restlessness and difficulty sleeping.

Put the day to bed – develop your own routine in the evening that allows you to wind down. This might involve watching TV if you find it relaxing, but avoid tuning in to anything that could prey on your mind later when you're trying to go to sleep, and always switch off at least half an hour before bed. Alternatively, try reading or listening to music.

Enjoy a warm bath before bedtime – your temperature rises with the warmth and then falls, helping you to drop off. The warmth can also ease muscular and mental tension, especially if you add relaxing essential oils like lavender or chamomile. Lavender has been shown to improve sleep quality by 20 per cent.

A small glass of wine could relax you – but large amounts of alcohol can disrupt sleep patterns and have diuretic effects, making you more likely to wake up and need the loo during the night. Cabernet Sauvignon, Merlot and Chianti are thought to promote sleep because they are made from grapes that are especially rich in melatonin.

Jot down any concerns or plans for the next day before bedtime – so that you don't lie awake worrying.

If you wake during the night and start mulling over problems – try telling yourself firmly: 'You can't do anything now, so go to sleep and think about it tomorrow.'

40. Manage migraines

A migraine is a debilitating, one-sided, pulsating headache. A study published in *Cephalagia* in 2006 involving 92 migraine sufferers – 72 women and 20 men – found that there was a higher incidence of fibromyalgia among the women. As well as the low serotonin link, another theory as to why fibromyalgia sufferers are likely to suffer from migraines, or vice versa, is that both conditions are linked to a hypersensitive central nervous system (the brain and nerves in the spinal column) that overreacts to external stimuli such as pain, light, noise, temperature, perfumes and chemicals; research published in *The Journal of Headache and Pain* reported that migraine and tension headache sufferers who also experience anxiety, sleep disturbance, and tenderness and pain on the outside of the head, are especially likely to develop fibromyalgia.

The two main types of migraine are migraine without aura, also known as 'common migraine' and migraine with aura, often called 'classical migraine'. Many people suffer from both types.

Classical migraines have four distinct stages. Common migraines have three.

Stages of migraine

Prodome – this starts up to 24 hours before an attack and is often characterised by a change in energy levels or mood, food cravings, excessive yawning or neck pain.

Aura (in classical migraines only) – is a sensory change, the most common of which is visual disturbance, such as blind spots, silvery starbursts, zigzag patterns or even tunnel vision, and can be frightening, especially when you first experience it. Other types of aura include pins and needles, and numbness down one side, speech disturbance, clumsiness and confusion.

Headache – this can last from four hours to three days and is accompanied by at least one of these other symptoms: nausea, vomiting, diarrhoea, increased sensitivity to light, sound or smell, lethargy and fatigue or a stiff, aching neck.

Recovery – this can take several days. It's common to feel tired and lacking in energy during this phase.

How can I prevent migraines?

A 'migraine brain' is hypersensitive to changes. These changes (usually known as triggers) can be anything from a drop in blood sugar from missing a meal, to changes in the weather or sleeping more or less than usual. Other triggers include hormonal changes, emotional stress, dehydration, exposure to bright or flickering lights and excessive exercise. Some people link their headaches to particular foods, such as cheese or chocolate, or to food additives, but experts argue that missing a meal is more likely to result in an attack than food intolerance. Alcohol – especially red wine – can be a trigger for some people.

Whatever your triggers are, it seems they upset the brain's chemistry, causing the blood vessels in the head to swell, which results in the all-too-familiar pain and other symptoms as parts of the brain effectively shut down. The best way to reduce the number of migraines you experience is to identify your own particular triggers; you can do this by keeping a migraine diary in which you record when each attack happens and details of your daily life at the time that might be relevant, e.g. food and drink, sleep and work patterns, stress levels, stage in menstrual cycle, etc. After a few weeks you should be able to pinpoint what triggers your attacks and, once you have done this, you can then aim to avoid them as much as possible. Bear in mind that often it isn't one particular trigger that causes an attack; usually a number of triggers have to occur before an individual's threshold is reached and a migraine develops.

Is there a cure for migraines?

There is no outright cure for migraines, but it is possible to prevent or at least reduce the number of attacks you have. Keeping to regular eating, drinking, sleeping, exercise, work and relaxation patterns as much as possible is the best way to avoid migraines. Eat a healthy, balanced diet and drink plenty of water to help avoid vitamin and mineral deficiencies and dehydration. Managing stress is important – yoga has been shown to help relieve stress and reduce the number and severity of migraine attacks.

Since fibromyalgia and migraines are both linked to low serotonin levels, 5-HTP (obtained from the Griffonia plant) might be a good supplement to try – see Chapter 5 – Benefit From Supplements. A lack of magnesium and B vitamins has also been linked with both fibromyalgia and migraines, so supplementing the diet with these nutrients may also help. There is evidence that other supplements, such as feverfew and butterbur, can also reduce the frequency and severity of attacks, and may be worth trying.

What's the best way to treat an attack?

Once an attack has started it's advisable to take painkillers as soon as you can, as the digestion slows down, making it harder for the body to absorb them. Many people find over-the-counter treatments such as aspirin, ibuprofen and paracetamol effective. Try taking your chosen medication alongside a cup of coffee or a glass of cola, as the caffeine in these drinks improves the effectiveness of the drugs and helps to constrict the swollen blood vessels. However, caffeine can be a migraine trigger for some.

If painkillers don't provide relief, you could try triptans. These work by balancing serotonin levels in the brain, which allows the blood vessels to return to normal. These are most effective when taken once the headache has started. There are several types; Imigran Recovery, which contains sumatriptan, is available over the counter on completion of a questionnaire to determine your suitability. Others, such as naratriptan, are available on prescription only.

Depending on the intensity of the attack, it's likely that you will need to rest, preferably in a quiet, darkened room, or wear an eye mask. A hot or cold compress on the site of the pain helps some people.

41. Ease IBS

Studies suggest that up to 70 per cent of people with fibromyalgia also suffer from IBS. Researchers are unsure why this is the case but, as well as low serotonin levels, other possible links include both conditions being associated with stress and also with disruption of normal muscle function; the gut is a 'smooth' muscle and IBS symptoms are caused by the gut, or part of it, being over-active – resulting in abdominal pain and diarrhoea – or under-active, leading to bloating, wind and constipation.

There are three types of IBS:

Alternating constipation and diarrhoea – IBS-A

Constipation predominant – IBS-C

Diarrhoea predominant – IBS-D

There is no cure, but it is possible to prevent attacks by identifying your triggers, and adapting your diet and lifestyle accordingly. A good way of discovering your triggers is to keep a record of your symptoms and any details that might be relevant, such as foods eaten, stress levels, stage in menstrual cycle, medications taken, etc. After a few weeks you should be able to pinpoint your individual triggers and then aim to avoid them as much as possible.

Adapt your diet

Many IBS sufferers notice a link between certain foods and their symptoms. Food triggers can include wheat, dairy products, citrus fruits, sugary, fatty or spicy foods, cabbage, onions and broccoli, and food additives. However, if you suspect a whole food group (e.g. dairy products or wheat) is causing your symptoms, seek advice from your GP or a dietician, who may suggest following an exclusion diet. This is best done under medical supervision to ensure you still follow a balanced diet – see Action 27 – Check for food intolerances for more information.

Altering the type and amount of fibre you eat according to your symptoms is probably the most effective dietary change you can make to ease IBS. There are two types of fibre: soluble, found in oats, barley, rye, vegetables, pulses and the fleshy part of fruits; and insoluble, found in wholegrain cereals, wholemeal bread, brown rice and pastas, and fruit and vegetable skins.

If you have IBS-A or IBS-D, try eating less insoluble fibre and more soluble fibre. Soluble fibre is less likely to irritate the gut lining. It's also less likely to lead to wind and bloating, because it's easily broken down.

If you have IBS-C, try eating more fibre and drinking more fluids. Do it gradually, as a sudden increase in fibre could lead to wind, bloating and diarrhoea. If this happens, try cutting down on foods containing insoluble fibre and eating more foods rich in soluble fibre to see if there is an improvement.

Kitchen cupboard remedies
Spices such as anise seed, cardamom pods and black pepper can aid digestion, and relieve wind and bloating.

Supplements that may help
Supplements that may help include: calcium to calm diarrhoea, magnesium to relieve constipation and probiotics to boost your 'good' bacteria levels.

Useful over-the-counter medications

Useful over-the-counter medications include:

◯ Colpermin and Mintec, which contain peppermint oil to dispel trapped wind.

◯ Buscopan, Fybogel Mebeverine, Colofac IBS and Spasmonal, which contain antispasmodics to relieve tummy cramps.

◯ Imodium and Diocalm Ultra, which ease diarrhoea by slowing down gut contractions.

Stress and IBS

Studies suggest a link between emotional stress and IBS so managing stress can help (see Chapter 2 – Pace Yourself, Rest and Relax). Self-hypnosis in particular has been shown to calm the gut.

42. Relieve restless legs syndrome (RLS)

A recent study found that fibromyalgia sufferers are 11 times more likely to suffer from restless legs syndrome (RLS). RLS is a type of sleep-related movement disorder where you have an irresistible urge to move your legs. Sufferers feel creeping sensations, sometimes accompanied by twitching, pain, tingling, itching or prickling which are temporarily relieved by moving the legs, but returns as soon as the legs are still again, making sleep difficult. The syndrome can be caused by iron-deficiency anaemia or folic acid deficiency and there may be a genetic link for some types. Some pregnant women suffer from the condition, especially in the last trimester of pregnancy.

The symptoms may also be linked to other underlying conditions such as diabetes, rheumatoid arthritis, neurological diseases or Parkinson's disease. Certain drugs can make RLS worse – these include antidepressants, calcium blockers, anti-nausea medications (not domperidone), some anti-allergy drugs and too much caffeine.

Dietary help

RLS may be helped by ensuring your diet contains adequate amounts of iron, folic acid and minerals, such as calcium, potassium and magnesium. Cutting back on stimulants like caffeine, nicotine and alcohol may also be beneficial. Staying well hydrated by drinking plenty of water often helps. Have a light, slow-release snack, such as oatcakes and low-fat cheese, or a yogurt, before going to bed to maintain blood sugar levels, as low blood sugar may play a part in RLS.

Supplementary benefits

Calcium and magnesium supplements may prevent cramping and twitching. Omega-3 fish oils, ginkgo biloba and garlic all help to boost circulation.

Get moving

Walking, stretching and yoga may also help to relieve the symptoms. If your leg movements are stopping you from sleeping, try massaging your legs or get up and walk around.

Other tips

Try putting hot or cold packs on your legs before going to bed. Over-the-counter painkillers such as ibuprofen and paracetamol can bring some relief.

43. Keep Raynaud's at bay

People suffering from fibromyalgia sometimes also experience Raynaud's phenomenon. During an attack the hands and feet become icy cold, as if they are inside a freezer, which makes carrying out basic tasks, such as cutting food, washing and dressing, or handling money, difficult. The condition affects the circulation in the extremities – usually the fingers and toes, but sometimes the nose and ears are affected. It happens when small blood vessels go into a temporary spasm in response to cold or stress. This causes the blood vessels to narrow, restricting the blood flow and causing the affected areas to turn white or blue. When the blood begins to flow again the affected areas turn red and there may be numbness, tingling and pain. It seems that sufferers are hypersensitive to changes in temperature and stress, which fits in with the theory that fibromyalgia is due to an oversensitive nervous system. The stress response naturally leads to blood vessels constricting, but in Raynaud's sufferers this reaction is exaggerated.

Prevent attacks

Avoid exposure to the cold as much as possible.

Wear layers of clothing in cold weather to help trap your body heat.

Wear gloves to keep your hands warm – including when you are getting food out of the fridge or freezer.

Be physically active to boost circulation and reduce stress.

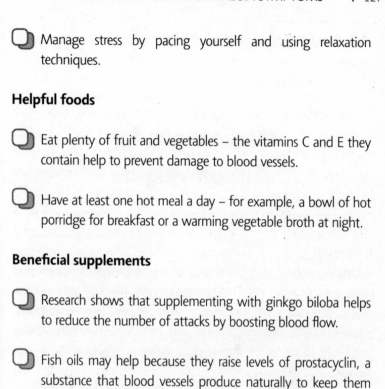

- Manage stress by pacing yourself and using relaxation techniques.

Helpful foods

- Eat plenty of fruit and vegetables – the vitamins C and E they contain help to prevent damage to blood vessels.

- Have at least one hot meal a day – for example, a bowl of hot porridge for breakfast or a warming vegetable broth at night.

Beneficial supplements

- Research shows that supplementing with ginkgo biloba helps to reduce the number of attacks by boosting blood flow.

- Fish oils may help because they raise levels of prostacyclin, a substance that blood vessels produce naturally to keep them dilated (widened) – but which Raynaud's sufferers are believed to lack.

Chapter 8

Medications for Fibromyalgia

If, despite making changes to your diet and lifestyle, the pain and other symptoms of fibromyalgia are severely affecting your quality of life, you may want to consider taking appropriate medications. However, both over-the-counter and prescribed medications can cause side effects so it is important to weigh up the benefits against the risks.

This chapter gives an overview of some of the over-the-counter and prescription-only medications commonly used for the relief of fibromyalgia symptoms, including painkillers and antidepressants, as well as newer drugs including an anticonvulsant and a dopamine agonist. It explains what the drugs are and how they work, as well listing potential side effects.

Not everyone will suffer side effects from taking medications and you may experience others in addition to those listed. You can report suspected side effects to MHRA online using their Yellow Card Scheme, or ask your GP or pharmacist to do so on your behalf.

Always read the leaflet that accompanies the medication and discuss any concerns with your pharmacist or GP before using it. Always inform your GP or pharmacist if you are taking any vitamin, mineral or herbal supplements, as these may interact with medications or reduce their effectiveness.

44. Find out about medications for fibromyalgia

Analgesics

What they are: Analgesics are painkillers. The over-the-counter drug paracetamol and the prescription-only drugs codeine and tramadol are the most commonly used painkillers for fibromyalgia.

What they do: Relieve pain.

How they work: Paracetamol blocks the production of hormone-like substances called prostaglandins in the brain and spinal cord, which make nerve endings more sensitive to pain. This means you feel less pain. Codeine blocks pain signals from the nerves to the brain. Tramadol reduces pain by boosting levels of serotonin in the nervous system.

Pros: Paracetamol is the cheapest and safest analgesic, as it doesn't irritate the stomach lining and generally has few side effects. Codeine is suitable for severe pain that isn't relieved by paracetamol. Tramadol not only relieves pain, but may also help improve your functioning in your daily activities.

Cons: Codeine can cause drowsiness, dizziness, nausea and constipation. Tramadol can cause nausea, constipation, diarrhoea and fatigue, and withdrawal symptoms if you stop taking it.

Cautions: Paracetamol is toxic to the liver, so overdosing is potentially very dangerous. It's important not to take more than one product containing paracetamol; remember that paracetamol is often included in cold and flu remedies and other preparations. If you are pregnant or breastfeeding, or have liver or kidney problems, let your GP or pharmacist know before you take paracetamol or codeine. If you have breathing, prostate or thyroid problems, or suffer from low blood pressure or epilepsy, let your GP or pharmacist know before you use codeine. If you want to stop taking tramadol do it gradually under your GP's supervision, as withdrawal symptoms can range from nervousness, panic, sweating, insomnia and numbness, pain, burning, or tingling in your hands or feet, to more severe symptoms such as uncontrollable shaking.

> If you suffer from constant pain you can take paracetamol throughout the day; the usual adult dose is two 500 mg tablets, four times a day. However, if you find that you need to take painkillers continuously over long periods it is worth reassessing your lifestyle to determine what is triggering your symptoms, and adopting appropriate preventative strategies such as exercise and relaxation.

Antidepressants

What they are: Antidepressants commonly used to treat fibromyalgia include the older tricyclic antidepressants (TCAs), such as amitriptyline and imipramine, and the newer serotonin-noradrenaline reuptake inhibitors (SNRIs) such as duloxetine, and selective serotonin reuptake inhibitors (SSRIs) such as fluoxetine and paroxetine.

What they do: Help to relieve pain and ease depression – although they are usually given in much lower doses for treating fibromyalgia;

you may be given a higher dose if you also have depression. They also improve sleep quality.

How they work: They boost levels of certain neurotransmitters, low levels of which are thought to be implicated in fibromyalgia. TCAs and SNRIs raise levels of serotonin and noradrenaline. SSRIs boost serotonin levels. Higher levels of these chemicals help to change the way the brain perceives pain.

Pros: These drugs are not thought to be addictive.

Cons: TCAs are linked to more severe side effects than SNRIs and SSRIs, such as difficulty urinating, dizziness, drowsiness, slowed reaction times, confusion, visual disturbances, tremors, weight gain and an irregular heartbeat. If you experience drowsiness or slowed reaction times you shouldn't drive or operate machinery. Possible side effects of SSRIs and SNRIs include nausea, low libido, blurred vision, diarrhoea or constipation, dizziness, dry mouth, loss of appetite, sweating, agitation and insomnia.

Cautions: Stopping TCAs abruptly can cause withdrawal symptoms, such as insomnia and increased dreaming, and flu-like symptoms including headache, sweating, chills, nausea or muscular aches. SSRIs should not be taken by anyone with a history of mania. They may increase the risk of suicidal thoughts in some people.

Other drugs used to treat fibromyalgia

Pregabalin
What it is: An anticonvulsant drug used to treat epilepsy, nerve pain and anxiety.

What it does: Helps to relieve pain and fatigue, and improve sleep.

How it works: Reduces the activity of the nerve cells that control the transmission of pain messages. With reduced pain, sleep improves and fatigue is relieved.

Pros: Pregabalin can help to improve fibromyalgia sufferers' overall well-being.

Cons: It can cause side effects such as dry mouth, dizziness, drowsiness and fatigue, poor concentration, constipation, nausea, vomiting, headache and weight gain.

Cautions: If you experience swelling of the lips, mouth or tongue, or shortness of breath, you may be suffering from an allergic reaction to pregabalin, and should go to the accident and emergency department of your nearest hospital immediately.

Pramipexole

What it is: A drug known as a dopamine receptor agonist, which is usually used to treat Parkinson's disease and restless legs syndrome.

What it does: Relieves pain and improves sleep.

How it works: It boosts dopamine levels. Dopamine is a neurotransmitter that reduces the body's response to pain.

Pros: Pramipexole also helps to relieve restless legs syndrome.

Cons: Common side effects include nausea, vomiting, constipation and headaches.

Cautions: Tell your GP if you start falling asleep suddenly, experience dizziness, fainting or hallucinations, or start behaving impulsively.

Muscle relaxants

What they are: Medications that relax the muscles, such as tizanidine (Zanaflex) and methocarbamol (Robaxin). They are usually prescribed for use at bedtime.

What they do: Relieve stiffness and spasms, help improve sleep and reduce fatigue.

How they work: They dampen down nerve signals to the muscles, which reduces muscle tension and any associated pain. This in turn improves sleep patterns.

Pros: Relieving stiffness can help to improve mobility.

Cons: Possible side effects include drowsiness, dizziness, headache, dry mouth, nausea, vomiting, diarrhoea and constipation, difficulty sleeping, hallucinations and a slower heart rate.

Cautions: Muscle relaxants should only be used in the short term for pain flare-ups. This drug can affect liver function. If you experience signs of jaundice (yellowing of the skin or the whites of the eyes) visit your GP or nearest accident and emergency department immediately.

Guaifenesin

What it is: An expectorant obtained from the guaiac tree, commonly found in cough medicines, and a controversial medication for fibromyalgia, discovered by fibromyalgia sufferer and US endocrinologist Dr Paul St Amand.

What it does: St Amand claims it relieves fibromyalgia symptoms.

How it works: St Amand believes that fibromyalgia is caused by excess calcium and phosphates being stored in the muscles, preventing them from producing energy. He claims that guaifenesin encourages the kidneys to excrete these substances through the urine, allowing the muscles to return to normal functioning.

Pros: Side effects from guaifenesin are uncommon.

Cons: A double-blind study in 1993 involving 40 fibromyalgia sufferers concluded that guaifenesin was no more effective than a placebo. St Amand argues that this is because the study did not warn participants to avoid salicylates found in medications, herbal remedies and topical products such as toiletries, cosmetics and mint toothpastes, all of which he claims blocks the effects of guaifenesin. Guaifenesin is not available in the UK on prescription, but can be bought online (see Useful Products).

Chapter 9

Try DIY Complementary Therapies

Complementary therapies (also known as alternative, natural or holistic therapies) focus on treating the whole person, as opposed to conventional Western medicine, which aims to treat the symptoms of ill health, rather than the individual. More and more people, concerned about side effects from prescribed drugs, are turning to complementary therapies to improve their general health, or to help them manage long-term health problems such as fibromyalgia.

Complementary therapy practitioners view illness as a sign that physical and mental well-being have been disrupted, and attempt to restore good health by stimulating the body's own self-healing and self-regulating abilities. They claim that total well-being comes from the mind and body being in a state of balance called homeostasis. Homeostasis can be achieved by following the type of lifestyle advocated in this book, i.e. a healthy diet with plenty of fresh air, exercise, sleep and relaxation, combined with stress management and a positive mental attitude. Complementary therapies such as aromatherapy, massage and reflexology can help you to achieve homeostasis on a physical and emotional level by improving sleep, relieving pain, reducing stress levels and promoting relaxation.

Whether complementary therapies work or not remains controversial. Some argue that any benefits of such therapies are due to the placebo effect; this is where a treatment improves symptoms simply because the person using it expects it to, rather than because it has any real effect. However, it could be argued that, unlike comparatively new drug treatments, complementary therapies have stood the test of time, having been used to treat ailments and promote well-being for thousands of years. The use of complementary therapies alongside conventional medicine received an unexpected boost recently when NICE recommended acupuncture and chiropractic treatments, along with exercise therapy, for the treatment of lower back pain.

This chapter gives you an overview of a selection of complementary therapies that may help to ease fibromyalgia – acupressure, the Alexander technique, aromatherapy, massage and homeopathy – including techniques and treatments you can try for yourself. Relevant useful organisations and products are listed in the Directory at the end of the book.

44. Apply acupressure

The use of acupressure for the treatment of fibromyalgia hasn't been evaluated; but acupressure is often described as 'acupuncture without needles' and some studies suggest that acupuncture can bring about short-term improvements in fibromyalgia symptoms, such as reduced pain and fewer tender points.

Like acupuncture, acupressure is part of traditional Chinese medicine and works on the same points on the body. Both are based on the idea that life energy, or *qi* (also referred to as 'chi'), flows through channels in the body known as meridians. An even passage of *qi* throughout the body is viewed as vital to good health. Disruption of the flow of *qi* in a meridian can lead to illness at any point within it. The flow of *qi* can be affected by various factors, including stress, emotional distress, diet and environment.

Qi is most concentrated at points along the meridians known as acupoints. There is some scientific evidence that stimulating specific acupoints can relieve pain. Practitioners claim that using the fingers and thumbs to apply firm but gentle pressure to these points stimulates the body's natural self-healing abilities. Muscular tension is relieved and circulation boosted, thereby promoting good health. The application of pressure is believed to stimulate the production of endorphins and encephalins (pain-relieving hormones), and to help to relax tense, taut muscles. Many Chinese people use acupressure to self-treat a range of common conditions. You can try the following simple acupressure techniques for yourself. For best results, press on the acupoint for about three minutes.

Shoulder well
To ease painful, stiff shoulders use your middle fingers to press firmly on both sides of the neck on the 'shoulder well' acupoints. These can be found half way down the slope between the neck and shoulders.

Third eye
To induce calm and aid sleep use both index fingers to apply firm pressure to the 'third eye' acupoint. This is located between the eyebrows, where the bridge of the nose joins the forehead.

The great energiser
To boost your energy levels, apply firm pressure to the 'great energiser' acupoints. The easiest way to do this is to fold your arms across your

chest with your left arm above your right arm. Now press into the end of the crease above the inside of your right elbow with your left thumb. Repeat on your left arm, using your right thumb.

45. Find relief with reflexology

The energy theory behind reflexology is very similar to the one underpinning acupressure, although practitioners say it is a different system.

Reflexology is based on the theory that points on the feet, hands and face, known as reflexes, correspond to specific parts of the body, including bones, glands, organs and muscles. They are linked via ten vertical zones, along which energy flows; these begin in the feet and hands and continue up to the head. If the energy flow within any of these zones becomes blocked illness may occur. Stimulating the reflexes using the fingers and thumbs is claimed to produce physiological changes that remove these blockages, and encourage the mind and body to self-heal.

Practitioners claim that imbalances in the body cause granular deposits in the relevant reflex, which result in tenderness. Corns, bunions and even hard skin are all believed to indicate problems in the related parts of the body. One small Icelandic study in 2010 into the effects of reflexology on pain and other symptoms in women with fibromyalgia, reported that a weekly reflexology treatment reduced pain in several parts of the body, including the head, neck and arms.

A reflexologist will usually work on your feet, because they believe the feet are more sensitive. However, it's usually much easier to work on your hands when you are self-treating. Below are three techniques that may help to relieve pain in the neck, shoulders and back, and involve using your thumbs to apply firm pressure to different parts of the hands.

Neck pain reliever

To relieve neck pain use your right thumb to creep around the base of your left thumb. Repeat several times and then carry out the same motions on your right hand, using your left thumb.

Shoulder pain reliever

To ease shoulder pain use your right thumb to creep up the centre of your little finger on your left hand, starting at the base and finishing at the tip. Repeat several times and then perform the same movements on your right hand, using your left thumb.

Back pain reliever

To relieve back pain creep your right thumb along the whole of the spinal reflex on the left hand. This begins in the middle of the inner wrist and extends right along the outside of the thumb to the tip. Repeat several times and then apply the same motions to your right hand using your left thumb.

46. Improve your posture with the Alexander technique

The Alexander technique is a useful discipline for fibromyalgia sufferers to learn, as it aims to improve posture and enable the body to function with the minimum amount of strain on the joints and muscles, helping to relieve muscular tension and pain. A study published in the *British Medical Journal* in 2008 reported that practising the Alexander technique provided significant long-term benefits for people with chronic back pain.

The technique was devised in the 1890s by Australian actor Frederick Matthias Alexander, after he realised he was tensing his muscles and adopting an unnatural posture in response to physical and emotional stress before a show, and that this was having a negative effect on his performance. Many of us are guilty of this – a common example is the irritation you feel when you are stuck in a traffic jam, and you unconsciously react to the situation by tightening your neck and shoulder muscles. Even brushing your teeth can cause unnecessary strain if you grasp the toothbrush too tightly, as this creates tension in the arm, shoulder and neck muscles. The Alexander technique teaches you to become aware of tension in your body, as well as your posture, movement and thinking, in order to overcome unhelpful habits, and it therefore encourages you to focus on living in the present.

According to practitioners, poor posture affects bone alignment, puts unnecessary stress on the joints, ligaments and muscles, and leads to pain. The Alexander technique focuses on restoring the correct positioning of the head, neck and back – 'the core' of the body – and the areas where the pain and tenderness of fibromyalgia are frequently felt. This involves learning how to free up the spine, neck and head, by imagining the spine and neck lengthening and softening, and allowing the head to rise up.

To ensure that you adopt the correct posture, it's best to learn the Alexander technique from a qualified teacher. A teacher will assess your posture and movement, and show you how to rectify any bad habits so that you can move more freely and naturally. You will learn how to perform everyday tasks such as turning on a tap with the minimum of force, to reduce strain on the muscles. Once you have become proficient you will be able to practise at home.

The long-term goal is for you to naturally hold your body in the correct stance all of the time.

However, in the meantime, here are three techniques you can try now:

Release muscular tension – first, identify which muscles are tense and mentally tell them to 'let go'. Imagine the tension melting away from the affected areas.

Stand up straight – hold your head up and distribute your weight evenly between your feet, unlock your knees, lengthen your spine, and free your neck and shoulder muscles. Your body weight should fall mainly on your heels.

Walk tall – adopt the standing position outlined above. As you walk, focus on your weight shifting from one foot to the other, making each movement as effortless as you can. Again, your heels should bear most of your weight.

47. Use aroma power

Essential oils are obtained using various methods from the petals, leaves, stalk, roots, seeds, nuts, and even the bark of plants. Aromatherapy is based on the belief that the inhalation of scents released from essential oils affects the hypothalamus – the part of the brain that controls the glands and hormones – altering mood and lowering stress. When used in massage, baths and compresses, the oils are also absorbed through the bloodstream, and carried to the organs and glands, which benefit from their healing effects. Since fibromyalgia flare-ups can be linked to emotional stress, aromatherapy may be worth trying, both as a preventative measure and during a flare-up.

Patricia Davies, author of *Aromatherapy: An A–Z*, recommends analgesic oils such as chamomile, lavender, marjoram, meadowsweet and rosemary to alleviate the pain of fibromyalgia.

Chamomile
The two main types of chamomile used in aromatherapy are Roman chamomile and German chamomile. Both types are soothing, calming and anti-inflammatory, and are good for relieving muscular aches and pains. A warm bath containing chamomile oil before bed can help to promote deep sleep.

Lavender
Lavender oil is especially beneficial for fibromyalgia because it not only relieves pain, but also promotes relaxation and sound sleep; Japanese researchers recently reported that it reduces the stress hormone cortisol. Inhaling lavender oil at bedtime has been shown to improve sleep quality by 20 per cent.

Marjoram
Marjoram has a warm, spicy scent. When used in massage, marjoram oil has a warming effect that eases pain and stiffness.

Meadowsweet
Meadowsweet oil contains salicylic acid, often known as 'nature's own aspirin' because aspirin is derived from it, making it excellent for relieving muscular pain. It is also anti-inflammatory and mildly sedative, making it helpful for insomnia.

Rosemary

Rosemary oil relieves muscular pain when used in massage, added to a warm bath or applied on a hot compress. It is also a brain stimulant, so it helps to boost concentration and has long been used to improve memory, making it ideal for fighting 'fibro-fog'.

Caution: Don't use rosemary at bedtime as its stimulant properties can exacerbate sleep problems. Rosemary should not be used by anyone with epilepsy, as it may trigger fits.

Aromatherapy techniques

These oils are effective for pain relief when used in a warm bath, as a hot compress or in massage (see Action 48 – massage away pain).

Take an aromatic bath

Fill the bath with comfortably hot water. When you are ready to get in, add six drops of your chosen essential oil. Stir the water with your hand to spread the oil, which will form a thin film on the water. The warmth from the water both aids absorption through the skin and releases aromatic vapours, which are inhaled.

Make a hot compress

Add four or five drops of essential oil to a basin of hot water and soak a facecloth or small towel in it. Wring out the excess moisture and place on the affected area.

48. Massage away pain

A study of 24 adults with fibromyalgia published in *The Journal of Rheumatology* in 2002 reported that massage improved sleep and mood, and reduced pain and the number of tender points. Research presented at the 2007 EFIC Pain Congress concluded that therapeutic massage was the most popular complementary therapy among fibromyalgia sufferers, due to its relaxing effects.

Whenever we feel pain, we automatically rub or massage the affected area. Massage involves touch – which can help to ease pain and stiffness, and reduce stress and tension. It's thought to work by promoting the release of endorphins (the body's own painkillers) and serotonin (a brain chemical involved in relaxation). It also reduces the level of stress hormones in the blood and boosts the circulation, helping to improve the removal of toxins from the body. As the muscles relax, pain and stiffness is relieved and mobility and flexibility improves.

However, it is important for both you and the person performing the massage to realise that the level of pressure you can tolerate will vary from day to day. Always tell the person giving the massage if you feel they are using too much pressure. Choose a firm, safe surface that is comfortable for both you and the massager – a chair, for example, or a towel on the floor with a cushion to support your head and neck.

Massage oil

In massage, a 2 per cent dilution is normally used: this equates to two drops per tsp of carrier oil. A carrier oil can be any vegetable oil, including good-quality olive or sunflower oil; almond, sesame or grapeseed oils are equally good. Never apply aromatherapy oils to broken skin and buy the best quality oils you can afford; like most things, you get what you pay for – cheaper oils may not be as pure as more expensive ones.

Ask a partner or friend to massage your painful areas, or try self-massage, using these basic techniques:

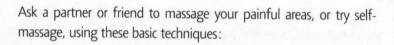 **Stroking/effleurage** – slide both hands over the skin in fanning or circular motions.

Kneading – using alternate hands, gently and rhythmically squeeze and release flesh between the fingers and thumbs, as if you're kneading dough.

Friction – using your thumbs, apply steady pressure to static points, or make tiny circles on each side of the spine.

Hacking – relax your hands; then, keeping your fingers apart, use the sides alternately to give short, sharp taps all over.

Playing some relaxing music in the background can help to enhance the feelings of relaxation.

Trigger point massage

Trigger point massage, or trigger point therapy as it is also known, involves using the stroking massage technique on trigger points – painful knotty areas that send pain elsewhere in the body when activated. Use slow movements in one direction only and limit the number of strokes to no more than 12 on each trigger point, up to 12 times daily. To gain the maximum benefit, you should apply enough pressure to make the area hurt a little, but on a scale of one to ten it should reach no more than seven, otherwise the muscles might contract even more in self-defence. Also be aware that it is likely to take a number of treatments to bring relief – especially if the trigger points are long established.

If you have trigger points in your back, shoulders and hips, but don't have anyone to massage them, or you can't manage to do it yourself, you could try using a tennis ball to release the knots. Trap the tennis ball between your body and another surface, for example, a wall, or a floor – depending on which you find easiest – so that it is applying pressure to the affected muscle. Again, you should expect to feel some pain, but it should not be unbearable. Warming the muscles first by having a hot shower or bath, or applying a heated pad or hot water bottle can help to relax the muscles and make them more receptive to the massage.

50. Get help with homeopathy

Homeopathy means 'same suffering' and is based on the belief that 'like cures like' – substances that can provoke symptoms in a well person can relieve the same symptoms in a person who is ill. For example, bee stings can cause hot, swollen, tender swellings, so the remedy apis, which is made from bee stings, is often prescribed for arthritis sufferers with swollen, tender joints.

Symptoms like inflammation or fever are seen as a sign that the body is trying to heal itself. The theory is that homeopathic remedies promote this self-healing process and that they work in a similar way to vaccines. The substances used in homeopathic remedies come from plant, animal, mineral, bark and metal sources. These substances are used to produce a tincture, which is then diluted many times over. Homeopaths claim that the more diluted a remedy is, the higher its potency and the lower its potential side effects. They believe in the 'memory of water', the theory that, even though the molecules from a substance are diluted, they leave behind an electromagnetic 'footprint' – rather like a recording on an audiotape – which has an effect on the body.

These ideas are controversial and many GPs remain sceptical; however, there is some evidence that homeopathy could help to ease fibromyalgia symptoms. A study of 30 fibromyalgia sufferers, at the Department of Rheumatology and Clinical Pharmacology at St Bartholomew's Hospital in London, reported that those taking the homeopathic remedy Rhus tox (see the following homeopathic remedies) had significantly bigger improvements in the number of tender points and overall quality of life. An RCT published in *Rheumatology* in 2004, involving 62 fibromyalgia sufferers with an average age of 49, concluded that those receiving an individually prescribed homeopathic remedy had significantly greater improvements in the number of tender points and pain, as well as quality of life, overall health and mood.

There are two main types of remedies – whole person based and symptom based. It's probably best to consult a qualified homeopath who will prescribe a remedy aimed at you as a whole person, based on your personality, as well as the symptoms you experience. However, if you prefer, you can buy homeopathic remedies at many high street pharmacies and health shops.

Below is a list of homeopathic remedies, along with the fibromyalgia-related symptoms for which they're used. To self-prescribe, simply choose the remedy with indications that most closely match your symptoms. Follow the dosage instructions on the product.

Arnica
Symptoms: Fibromyalgia brought on by an accident or traumatic event; pain that feels like bruising and is worse when you touch the affected area.

Bryonia
Symptoms: Tight muscles and pain that worsens with movement and warmth; headaches and irritability.

Causticum
Symptoms: Sore, weak, stiff muscles that are worse when overused or it is cold, and better with warmth; tight, sore leg muscles and restlessness at night.

Cimicifuga
Symptoms: Muscular spasms, jerking and twitching and feeling sore and bruised all over. Pain – mainly in the back, neck and shoulders – that improves in warmth.

Gelsemium
Symptoms: Heavy limbs, headaches and dizziness. Symptoms are worse after exertion and in cold, damp weather.

Hypericum
Symptoms: Nerve pain, especially prickly pain, numbness, or tingling; pain that is worse with movement and when affected area is touched; also beneficial for fibromyalgia-related depression.

Rhus tox
Symptoms: Pain and stiffness that worsens when you first start moving around and improves with heat; restlessness and impatience.

Not a quick fix

Practitioners warn that homeopathy isn't a 'quick fix' – the remedies may take a while to work. Homeopathic remedies are generally considered safe and don't have any known side effects, although sometimes a temporary worsening of symptoms known as 'aggravation' may take place. This is seen as a good sign, as it suggests that the remedy is stimulating the healing process. If this happens, stop taking the remedy and wait for your symptoms to improve. If there is steady improvement, don't restart the remedy. If the improvement stops, resume taking the remedy.

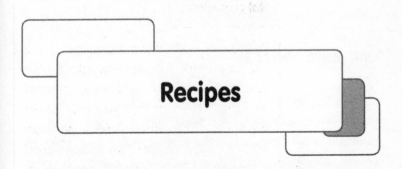

Recipes

This section features recipes based on some of the dietary recommendations outlined in this book. All of the dishes are not only nutritious, but also quick and easy to prepare.

Muesli (serves 2)

In this recipe the oats, almonds and seeds boost serotonin levels and supply magnesium and omega-3 fats. The dried fruits provide vitamins and soluble fibre.

Ingredients
100 g rolled oats
25 g dried apricots, chopped
25 g raisins
25 g whole almonds
1 tbsp pumpkin seeds
1 tbsp sunflower seeds
Milk or yogurt to serve

Method
Mix together the oats, dried apricots, raisins, whole almonds, pumpkin seeds and sunflower seeds in a large bowl, then spoon into

a serving bowl. Serve with semi-skimmed or skimmed milk, or low-fat natural or Greek yogurt.

Tuna pasta (serves 2)

In this recipe the tuna helps to boost serotonin levels, while the wholewheat pasta balances the blood sugar. The garlic, basil and olive oil are anti-inflammatory and the tomatoes, onions and peppers provide antioxidants. The Parmesan cheese is a good source of protein, calcium, zinc, vitamin A and vitamins B2 and B12.

Ingredients
160 g of wholegrain spaghetti/pasta twists
3 tbsp of olive oil
1 red pepper, cut into 1 cm pieces
1 red onion, chopped
100 g cherry/plum tomatoes
150 g can of tuna in spring water
50 g Parmesan cheese, shaved
1 clove garlic, finely chopped
½ red chilli, chopped
6 fresh basil leaves, torn

Method
Cook pasta according to the instructions on the packet. Heat the olive oil in frying pan. Add the pepper and onion and stir-fry gently until it begins to soften, then add the cherry/plum tomatoes, garlic and chilli. Continue to fry until all of the ingredients in the pan are soft.

Stir the cooked vegetables into the cooked pasta. Mix in the drained tuna and torn basil leaves. Place on serving plate. Sprinkle with the Parmesan cheese shavings.

Pan-fried lamb's liver with sweet potato mash and red wine gravy (serves 1)

In this recipe the liver provides protein and B vitamins, along with the sweet potato, supplies useful amounts of vitamins A and D, while the olive oil provides monounsaturated fats and is anti-inflammatory.

Ingredients

For the liver
2 tbsp plain flour
Salt and freshly ground black pepper
100 g lamb's liver
1 tbsp olive oil

For the mash
½ sweet potato, peeled and cubed
15 g olive oil/olive margarine

For the gravy
1 tbsp olive oil
½ onion, sliced
50 ml red wine
200 ml boiling water
Handful chopped fresh chives, to serve

Method

Sprinkle the flour onto a plate with a little salt and freshly ground black pepper. Coat the liver in the mixture. Heat the oil in a frying pan over a medium heat. Fry the floured lamb's liver until crisp and golden-brown on both sides (about 2–3 minutes). Remove from the pan and set aside on a warm plate. Bring a pan of water to the boil, add sweet potato and cook until soft. Drain well, add olive oil or olive margarine and mash with a potato masher. Season to taste with a little salt and freshly ground black pepper. To make the gravy, heat the olive oil in the pan the liver was cooked in. Add the onion and fry until softened (about 5–6 minutes). Add the red wine, stirring well. Add the boiling water, reduce the heat and simmer until gravy has thickened (about 6–8 minutes). To serve, slice the liver in two. Pile the mash into the middle of a serving plate then put the liver on top. Pour the gravy around the edge of the plate and garnish with the chopped chives.

Smoked mackerel, cherry tomato and rocket salad (serves 4)

In this dish the mackerel is a great source of anti-inflammatory omega-3 fats, protein and vitamin D. The rocket is rich in vitamin B9 (folic acid/folate) and the tomatoes provide vitamins A and C and other phytonutrients (plant nutrients) with antioxidant properties, such as lycopene and lutein.

Ingredients
4 cooked smoked mackerel fillets
450 g cherry tomatoes, halved
70 g wild rocket
Freshly ground black pepper to taste
3–4 tbsp extra virgin oil/rapeseed oil
Juice of ½ a lemon

Method
Put the tomatoes into a bowl and toss with black pepper. Add the wild rocket and toss together once more. Whisk together the olive oil and lemon juice in a bowl. Heap the salad into the middle of

four plates. Place the mackerel fillet on top and drizzle with the olive oil and lemon juice dressing. Serve straight away with granary or wholemeal bread.

Greek plums (serves 2)

In this recipe the plums provide vitamins A and C, other antioxidants and insoluble fibre, while the Greek yogurt also provides vitamin A, as well as protein, calcium and beneficial bacteria.

Ingredients
250 ml water
3 tbsp honey
1 tsp ground cinnamon
12 plums
150 g low-fat Greek yogurt

Method
Put the water, cinnamon and honey into a pan and heat, stirring until the honey has dissolved.

Simmer gently for 5 minutes before adding the plums. Simmer for 5 more minutes or until the plums are soft. Remove from the heat. Serve the warm plums on a bed of Greek yogurt, with a drizzle of the syrup.

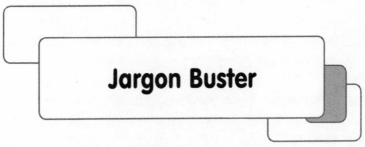

Jargon Buster

Below are explanations of medical terms in this book.

Autoimmune response – where the immune system mistakes normal tissues for foreign invaders and attacks them, giving rise to autoimmune diseases such as rheumatoid arthritis.

Cortisol – a hormone released by the adrenal glands during the stress response.

Endorphins – the body's own painkillers.

Free radicals – substances produced by normal chemical reactions in the body and linked to cell damage.

Glycaemic index – a ranking of foods according to the effect they have on blood sugar levels.

Inflammation – the immune system's natural response to irritation, infection, or injury; symptoms include redness, heat, swelling and pain.

Ligament – tissue that connects one bone to another.

Osteoarthritis – a condition generally caused by wear and tear of the joints that leads to pain, stiffness and inflammation.

Rheumatoid arthritis – an autoimmune disease characterised by swollen, painful joints.

Salicylates – plant hormones commonly found in foods, medications like aspirin, herbal remedies, cosmetics and toiletries.

Serotonin – a neurotransmitter involved in pain regulation, mood, appetite and sleep.

Tendon – tissue that connects muscle to bone.

Trigger point – tense knotted muscle that transfers pain to other parts of the body when 'activated'.

Tryptophan – an amino acid the body uses to make serotonin.

Helpful Books

Craggs-Hinton, Christine, *Living with Fibromyalgia* (Sheldon Press, 2010). This book provides an overview of fibromyalgia, and covers various aspects, including medications, diet, posture and exercise. The author herself suffers from fibromyalgia.

Davies, Clair and Davies, Amber, *The Trigger Point Therapy Workbook: Your Self-Treatment Guide for Pain Relief* (New Harbinger Publications, 2004). A comprehensive guide to trigger point therapy and how to treat yourself using trigger point massage.

Davis, Patricia, *Aromatherapy – An A-Z* (Vermillion, 2005). A useful introduction to essential oils and how to use them to relieve stress and improve your well-being.

Ingham, Penny, *The Well-Tuned Body: Banish Back Pain With Gentle Exercises Based on the Alexander Technique* (Summersdale, 2006). A practical introduction to the Alexander technique, written by a professional Alexander technique teacher. The book explains how to recognise tension in your body and how to sit and stand correctly to help alleviate neck, shoulder and back pain.

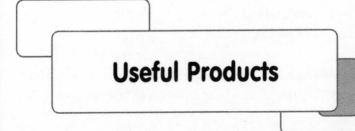

Useful Products

Below is a list of products and suppliers of products that may help to ease the symptoms of fibromyalgia. The author doesn't endorse or recommend any particular product and this list is by no means exhaustive.

Bio Care Magnesium Malate 90 Vegicaps
Capsules providing 720 mg of malic acid and 116.7 mg of magnesium.
Website: www.bodykind.com

CherryActive
A range of products containing red Montmorency cherries, which are rich in antioxidants and melatonin, to help relieve pain and promote sound sleep.
Website: www.cherryactive.co.uk

G Baldwin & Co
Herbalist founded in London in 1844. Offers a wide range of herbal supplements, tinctures and tea bags.
Website: www.baldwins.co.uk

Happy Days 100 mg 5-HTP

Supplement containing 100 mg of 5-HTP, vitamin C, biotin, niacin, vitamin B6, folic acid and zinc.

Website: www.healthspan.co.uk

HealthAid Sibergin 2500 Siberian Ginseng

Capsules containing 2,500 mg of concentrated Siberian Ginseng root extract.

Website: www.healthaid.co.uk

HealthAid Siberian Ginseng Liquid

Herbal liquid derived from organically grown herbs. Taken in a small amount of warm water.

Website: www.healthaid.co.uk

Herbs for Healing

A Gloucester-based company with an online shop selling medicinal plants and dried herbs, as well as herbal bath and skin products, and the equipment and ingredients to make your own. The website also offers useful information about the medicinal properties of herbs and herbal recipes.

Website: www.herbsforhealing.net

Holland & Barrett Complete B Vitamin B Complex Caplets

Caplets providing seven different B vitamins.

Website: www.hollandandbarrett.com

Holland & Barrett 5-HTP Capsules (50 mg)

Capsules containing 50 mg of 5-HTP from Griffonia seed extract.

Website: www.hollandandbarrett.com

Holland & Barrett Sunvite Vitamin D3 Caplets (25 mcg)

Caplets containing 25 mcg (1,000 IU) of vitamin D.
Website: www.hollandandbarrett.com

Kira Good Mood St John's Wort Extract 450 mg

A traditional herbal supplement containing standardised 450 mg of St John's wort extract.
Website: www.thehealthcounter.com

Large Multi-Purpose Wheat Bag

Pillow measuring 34 cm x 19 cm that contains wheat and lavender, and can be heated in the microwave to provide relief from pain. Available in three colours.
Website: www.ease-pain.com

Lifeplan Siberian Ginseng (600 mg)

Tablets containing 600 mg of Siberian ginseng. Free from added sugar, salt, starch, lactose, gluten, live yeasts, synthetic flavours, artificial colours or preservatives. Suitable for vegans.
Website: www.lifeplan.co.uk

Nature's Best Pure Grade St John's Wort High Strength One-a-Day

Tablets containing 340 mg of concentrated St John's wort extract.
Website: www.naturesbest.co.uk

Nelson's Homeopathic Pharmacy

Online retailer selling homeopathic remedies, including a combination for nervous anxiety that includes Arsen alb, aconite and gelsemium. Also sells Bach flower remedies.
Website: www.nelsonshomeopathy.com

Prewett's Instant Chicory (100 g)

A caffeine-free alternative to coffee, made from roasted chicory root.
Website: www.healthstore.uk.com

Probio 7 Advanced Formula

Maximum-strength probiotic capsules to rebalance gut bacteria, protect against bloating and diarrhoea, and boost immunity.
Website: www.hollandandbarrett.com

Pro Health Guaifenesin Fast Acting (400 mg)

Fast-acting capsules containing 400 mg guaifenesin.
Website: www.yourhealthbasket.co.uk

SAMe 400 mg enteric coated tablets by Biovea

Tablets containing 400 mg of SAMe, suitable for vegans.
Website: www.biovea.co.uk

Seven Seas Pure Cod Liver Oil

10 ml (2 tsp) provides 400 IU of vitamin D, 828 mg of EPA and 736 mg DHA (omega-3 fatty acids).
Website: www.seven-seas.com

Solgar Formula Vitamin B-Complex '100' Tablets

High-potency tablets containing vitamin B complex.
Website: www.solgar.co.uk

Solgar Siberian Ginseng Root Extract

Contains powdered Siberian ginseng root and powder, and standardised root extract.
Website: www.solgar.co.uk

Solgar Vitamin D3 Softgels 1,000 IU
Softgel capsules containing 1,000 IU of vitamin D from fish liver oils.
Website: www.solgar.co.uk

The Stick Original Body Stick (blue handles)
A pole with spindles for deep-tissue massage.
Website: www.the-stick.co.uk

Symingtons Classic Dandelion Coffee (100 g)
Caffeine-free coffee substitute made from dandelion roots.
Website: www.healthstore.uk.com

Tisserand Aromatherapy Pure Essential Oils
A wide range of good-quality essential oils designed to improve health and happiness.
Website: www.tisserand.com

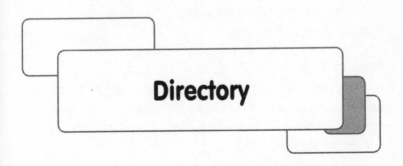

Directory

Below is a list of contacts offering useful information, support and services for fibromyalgia sufferers.

ABC of Yoga
A website offering tips, advice and poses for those who wish to practise yoga at home. Also provides meditation techniques.
Website: www.abc-of-yoga.com

Accessible Travel
A travel company that specialises in providing holidays both in the UK and abroad that are especially tailored to the needs of people with disabilities, including mobility problems.
Address: Avionics House, Kingsway Business Park, Naas Lane, Quedgeley, Gloucester GL2 2SN
Telephone: 01452 729739
Email: info@accessibletravel.co.uk
Website: www.accessibletravel.co.uk

The American Fibromyalgia Syndrome Association
A leading US medical charity dedicated to funding research that accelerates the pace of medical discoveries to improve the quality of

life for patients with fibromyalgia. The website offers information on fibromyalgia based on the latest research.
Website: www.afsafund.org

Arthritis Care

A UK charity that primarily offers self-help support to arthritis sufferers but also provides up-to-date information on fibromyalgia.
Address: Arthritis Care, 18 Stephenson Way, London NW1 2HD
Telephone: 020 7380 6500
Helpline (freephone): 0808 800 4050
Email: info@arthritiscare.org.uk
Website: www.arthritiscare.org.uk

Arthritis Research UK

As well as funding research, this UK charity produces a range of free information booklets and leaflets not only about arthritis but also fibromyalgia.
Address: Arthritis Research UK, PO Box 177, Chesterfield, Derbyshire S41 7TQ
Telephone: 0870 850 5000
Website: www.arthritisresearchuk.org

The British Pain Society

An alliance of medical professionals whose aim is to advance the understanding and management of pain. The website offers up-to-date information on pain management, including downloadable leaflets on understanding and managing pain, and downloadable copies of *Pain News*, the organisation's quarterly newsletter.
Address: The British Pain Society, Third Floor, Churchill House, 35 Red Lion Square, London WC1R 4SG
Telephone: 020 7269 7840
Email: info@britishpainsociety.org
Website: www.britishpainsociety.org

DIAL UK
A UK charity run by and for disabled people, with a network of disability information and advice line services (DIALs) offering advice on all aspects of living with a disability.
Address: St Catherine's, Tickhill Road, Doncaster, South Yorkshire DN4 8QN
Telephone: 01302 310123
Website: www.dialuk.info

Disabled Living Foundation (DLF)
A national charity that provides impartial advice, information and training on everyday living aids.
Address: 380–384 Harrow Road, London W9 2HU
Telephone: 020 7289 6111
Helpline: 0845 130 9177
Website: www.dlf.org.uk

FibroAction
A charity that offers information and support to people with fibromyalgia.
Helpline: 0844 443 5422
Email: info@fibroaction.org
Website: www.fibroaction.org

Fibromyalgia Association Scotland (FMA Scotland)
A charity dedicated to providing information, advice and support to people who suffer with fibromyalgia in Scotland. Members receive a quarterly newsletter.
Website: www.fmascotland.org.uk

Fibromyalgia Association UK

Fibromyalgia Association UK is a registered charity run by unpaid volunteers to promote greater awareness and education about fibromyalgia to sufferers and their families and medical professionals. Other services include national helplines on fibromyalgia and benefits, support groups across the UK and an online support forum.

Address: Training and Enterprise Centre, Applewood Grove, Cradley Heath B64 6EW

National helpline: 0844 887 2444 (10 a.m.–4 p.m. Mon–Fri)

Benefits helpline: 0844 887 2450 (10 a.m.–12 p.m. Mon and Fri)

Email: Complete online contact form on website.

Website: www.fmauk.org

Fibromyalgia Coalition International

A US charity that aims to give hope to everyone suffering from fibromyalgia and chronic fatigue syndrome, through research and the provision of information on natural, proven and effective therapies that focus on the root causes. You can also subscribe to the charity's quarterly *Fibromyalgia Alternative News* and the *Conquering the Challenge* newsletter.

Website: www.fibrocoalition.org

Fibromyalgia.com

US website that offers information and support to fibromyalgia sufferers.

Website: www.fibromyalgia.com

Fibromyalgia Network

A US organisation that provides support and information for fibromyalgia sufferers. Members also receive the quarterly *Fibromyalgia Network Journal* and monthly email alerts.

Website: www.fmnetnews.com

Fibromyalgia Support Net

A website founded by the husband of a fibromyalgia sufferer that sets out to make finding information about fibromyalgia quick and easy.

Email: Complete contact form online.

Website: www.fibromyalgia-support.net

Fibromyalgia Support N. Ireland

Fibromyalgia Support N. Ireland (FMSNI) is a non-profit-making organisation dedicated to providing help, information and support for fibromyalgia sufferers in the UK and Ireland, and those who care for them. Members receive a quarterly newsletter.

Helpline: 0844 826 9024 (national rates apply)

Website: www.fmsni.org.uk

Fibromyalgia Support Resource

US website that aims to keep fibromyalgia sufferers up to date with current news on research and treatment. Also provides message boards, chat rooms and a newsletter.

Website: www.fibromyalgiasupport.com

Fibromyalgia Syndrome

A website designed to help support people with fibromyalgia, and their families, friends and colleagues, by providing up-to-date information about fibromyalgia syndrome.

Website: www.fibromyalgiasyndrome.co.uk

Health Unlocked

A website that aims to gather the knowledge and experience of patients and to share it with others via online communities. Members' feedback suggests that the information and sense of support can reduce the isolation and fear experienced by people with chronic conditions.

Website: www.healthunlocked.com

Medicines and Healthcare products Regulatory Agency (MHRA)

A government agency responsible for ensuring that medicines and medical devices work, and are acceptably safe.

Address: Market Towers, 1 Nine Elms Lane, London SW8 5NQ

Telephone: 020 7084 2000/020 7210 3000

Email: info@mhra.gsi.gov.uk

Website: www.mhra.gov.uk

National Fibromyalgia & Chronic Pain Association

A US charity that works to provide information and support for people who have chronic pain conditions, as well as their families and friends. Members receive copies of the organisation's newsletter, bi-monthly magazine (digital or print version) and regular emails.

Website: www.fmcpaware.org

The National Fibromyalgia Partnership

A US not-for-profit educational organisation, offering medically accurate information on the symptoms, diagnosis, treatment of and research into fibromyalgia.

Website: www.fmpartnership.org

The National Fibromyalgia Research Association

US association that describes itself as a 'fibromyalgia syndrome (FMS) activist organisation in Salem, Oregon', that is dedicated to education, treatment and finding a cure for fibromyalgia. The website offers up-to-date information and details of the latest research.

Website: www.nfra.net

Pain Relief Foundation

A UK charity dedicated to funding research and education into the relief of chronic pain in humans. The website offers information about conditions which feature chronic pain, such as fibromyalgia.

Address: The Pain Relief Foundation, Clinical Sciences Centre, University Hospital Aintree, Lower Lane, Liverpool L9 7AL

Telephone: 0151 529 5820

Email: administrator@painrelieffoundation.org.uk

Website: www.painrelieffoundation.org.uk

PainSupport

A website offering pain relief techniques for those suffering from chronic pain. There is also a regular email newsletter, a discussion forum and a contact club for making new friends.

Email: Complete online contact form.

Website: www.painsupport.co.uk

Patient.co.uk

A website that offers 'comprehensive health information as provided by GPs and nurses to patients during consultations'. It also provides discussion forums where you can read about and share experiences of medical conditions, including fibromyalgia and relevant medications, treatments and services.

Website: www.patient.co.uk/forums

Select Food

An online directory of companies selling foods for people with allergies, such as dairy-, wheat-, gluten- and nut-free products.

Email: info@selectfood.co.uk

Website: www.selectfood.co.uk

The Soap Kitchen Warehouse

Online shopping site that sells a range of ingredients from which you can make your own cleaning products, such as borax, bicarbonate of soda and essential oils.

Website: www.soapkitchenonline.co.uk

The Society of Teachers of the Alexander Technique (STAT)

Website that provides information about the Alexander technique, including the latest research, a database of Alexander technique teachers, and details of courses and workshops across the UK.

Address: 1st Floor, Linton House, 39–51 Highgate Road, London NW5 1RS

Telephone: 0845 230 7828

Website: www.stat.org.uk

UK Fibromyalgia

A UK charity that offers up-to-date information about fibromyalgia online, as well as an online forum and details of a network of support groups across the UK. It also publishes a print and digital version of *The Fibromyalgia Magazine* each month, which covers various topics of interest to fibromyalgia sufferers, including medical research, legal and benefits advice, news from support groups, alternative therapies and pain management, as well as a separate email newsletter.

Address: 7 Ashbourne Road, Bournemouth, Dorset BH5 2JS

Email: info@ukfibromyalgia.com

Telephone/fax: 01202 259155

Website: www.ukfibromyalgia.com

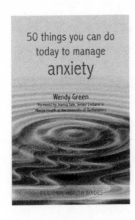

50 things you can do today to manage anxiety

Wendy Green
Foreword by Joanne Sale, Senior Lecturer in Mental Health at the University of Bedfordshire

PERSONAL HEALTH GUIDES

50 THINGS YOU CAN DO TODAY TO MANAGE ANXIETY

Wendy Green

ISBN: 978-1-84953-039-2

Paperback   £6.99

In this easy-to-follow book, Wendy explains how psychological, genetic and dietary factors can contribute to anxiety and offers practical advice and a holistic approach to help you deal with the symptoms, including simple dietary and lifestyle changes and DIY complementary therapies. Find out 50 things you can do today including:

- ○ Replace negative thoughts and behaviour with positive ones
- ○ Manage stress and relax to reduce symptoms
- ○ Choose beneficial foods and supplements
- ○ Find helpful organisations and products

'A very useful resource... offers people who are suffering from anxiety clear and current information and approaches... easy to follow, in particular during periods of anxiety or panic'
    Joanne Sale, senior lecturer in mental health, University of Bedfordshire

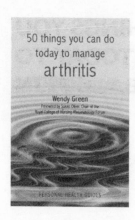

50 THINGS YOU CAN DO TODAY TO MANAGE ARTHRITIS

Wendy Green

ISBN: 978-1-84953-054-5

Paperback **£6.99**

In this easy-to-follow book, Wendy explains how genetics, age, infections, diet, excess weight, previous injuries and stress contribute to arthritis and offers practical advice and a holistic approach to help you deal with the symptoms, including simple dietary and lifestyle changes and DIY complementary therapies. Find out 50 things you can do today including:

° Choose beneficial foods and supplements
° Manage stress and relax to prevent and ease pain
° Discover practical tips to make everyday living easier
° Identify ways to help young arthritis sufferers
° Find helpful organisations and products

'an excellent resource for anyone who wishes to take some control over their arthritis… The author balances all the information for you in a quick and easy format'

Susan Oliver, nurse advisor to the National Rheumatoid Arthritis Society

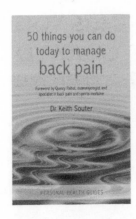

50 THINGS YOU CAN DO TODAY TO MANAGE BACK PAIN

Keith Souter

ISBN: 978-1-84953-120-7

Paperback £6.99

In this easy-to-follow book, Dr Keith Souter explains the various types and the many possible causes of back pain and offers practical and holistic advice to help you deal with it. With many years' experience as a GP, medical acupuncturist and homoeopathic specialist he looks at lifestyle changes, dietary modification and DIY complementary therapies that help to reduce back pain. Find out 50 things you can do today including:

○ Choose beneficial foods and supplements
○ Discover natural anti-inflammatory herbs and spices
○ Try out exercises to reduce pain and strengthen the back
○ Find helpful organisations and products

'clear, splendidly informative and well-thought-out… all the information you need in your journey towards a good, healthy and functional back'
Quincy Rabot, osteomyologist and specialist in
back pain and sports medicine

Have you enjoyed this book?
If so, why not write a review on your favourite website?

If you're interested in finding out more about our non-fiction
books follow us on Twitter: **@Summersdale**

Thanks very much for buying this Summersdale book.

www.summersdale.com